Research Advances in Genetics and Genomics

Implications for Psychiatry

Research Advances in Genetics and Genomics

Implications for Psychiatry

Edited by

Nancy C. Andreasen, M.D., Ph.D.

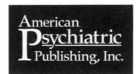

Washington, DC
London, England

Copyright © 2005 American Psychiatric Publishing, Inc.
ALL RIGHTS RESERVED

Manufactured in the United States of America on acid-free paper
09 08 07 06 05   5 4 3 2 1
First Edition

Typeset in Adobe's Palatino and Frutiger 55 Roman

American Psychiatric Publishing, Inc.
1000 Wilson Boulevard
Arlington, VA 22209-3901
www.appi.org

Unless otherwise noted, the articles contained in this volume are reprinted from *The American Journal of Psychiatry*, Volume 160, Number 4, April 2003. Chapter 2, "Psychiatric Genetics," is reprinted from *The American Journal of Psychiatry*, Volume 162, Number 1, January 2005.

Library of Congress Cataloging-in-Publication Data
Research advances in genetics and genomics : implications for
psychiatry / edited by Nancy C. Andreasen.— 1st ed.
      p. ; cm.
   Selected articles reprinted from v. 160, April 2003, of the American
journal of psychiatry.
   Includes bibliographical references and index.
   ISBN 1-58562-200-1 (pbk. : alk. paper)
   1. Mental illness—Genetic aspects. 2. Behavior genetics. 3. Genomics.
4. Human genetics. I. Andreasen, Nancy C.
   [DNLM: 1. Mental Disorders—genetics. 2. Genetics. 3. Genomics.
4. Psychiatry—methods. WM 140 R429 2005]
RC455.4.G4R47 2005
616.89′042—dc22

                                                                    2004055397

British Library Cataloguing in Publication Data
A CIP record is available from the British Library.

Contents

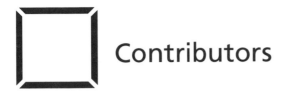

Contributors

Huda Akil, Ph.D.
Co-Director and Research Professor, Mental Health Research Institute, University of Michigan, Ann Arbor, Michigan

Nancy C. Andreasen, M.D., Ph.D.
Andrew H. Woods Chair of Psychiatry, University of Iowa College of Medicine, Iowa City, Iowa; Director, The MIND Institute, Albuquerque, New Mexico; Editor-In-Chief, *The American Journal of Pyshiatry*

Blynn G. Bunney, Ph.D.
Specialist, Department of Psychiatry, University of California, Irvine, California

William E. Bunney, M.D.
Della Martin Chair of Psychiatry, Department of Psychiatry, University of California, Irvine, California

Prabhakara V. Choudary, Ph.D.
Adjunct Professor, Center for Neuroscience, University of California, Davis, California

Francis S. Collins, M.D., Ph.D.
Director, National Human Genome Research Institute, National Institutes of Health, Bethesda, Maryland

Simon J. Evans, Ph.D.
Research Investigator, Department of Psychiatry, University of Michigan, Ann Arbor, Michigan

Irving I. Gottesman, Ph.D., Hon. F.R.C.Psych.
Professor of Psychiatry, Department of Psychiatry, University of Minnesota Medical School, Minneapolis, Minnesota

Todd D. Gould, M.D.
Research Fellow, Laboratory of Molecular Pathophysiology, Mood and Anxiety Disorders Program, National Institute of Mental Health, Bethesda, Maryland

Thomas R. Insel, M.D.
Director, National Institute of Mental Health and the National Human Genome Research Institute, Bethesda, Maryland

Edward G. Jones, M.D., Ph.D.
Director, Center for Neuroscience, University of California, Davis, California

Kenneth S. Kendler, M.D.
Professor of Psychiatry and Human Genetics and Director, Psychiatric Genetics, Virginia Institute for Psychiatry and Behavioral Genetics and the Departments of Psychiatry and Human Genetics, Medical College of Virginia of Virginia Commonwealth University, Richmond, Virginia

Jun Li, Ph.D.
Senior Scientist, Department of Genetics, Stanford University School of Medicine, Stanford, California

Kathleen Ries Merikangas, Ph.D.
Chief, Section on Developmental Genetic Epidemiology, Mood and Anxiety Disorders Program, National Institute of Mental Health, Bethesda, Maryland

Richard M. Myers, Ph.D.
Professor of Genetics, Stanford University, Stanford, California

Marshall Nirenberg, Ph.D.
National Institutes of Health, Chief of the Laboratory of Biochemical Genetics, National Heart, Lung, and Blood Institute, Bethesda, Maryland

Neil Risch, Ph.D.
Professor of Genetics, Department of Genetics, Stanford University School of Medicine, Stanford, California

Laurence H. Tecott, M.D., Ph.D.
Professor of Psychiatry, Department of Psychiatry, University of California, San Francisco, California

Hiroaki Tomita, Ph.D.
Assistant Researcher, Department of Psychiatry, University of California, Irvine, California

Marquis P. Vawter, Ph.D.
Assistant Researcher, Department of Psychiatry, University of California, Irvine, California

James D. Watson, Ph.D.
Chancellor, Cold Spring Harbor Laboratory, Cold Spring Harbor, New York

Stanley J. Watson, M.D., Ph.D.
Co-Director and Research Professor, Mental Health Research Institute, University of Michigan, Ann Arbor, Michigan

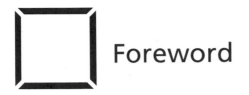

Foreword

The Double Helix 50 Years Later: Implications for Psychiatry

Fifty years ago, we knew the "double helix" was a pivotal discovery, despite the studied understatement with which we concluded our paper in *Nature*. But even we did not anticipate the richness and diversity of the discoveries that would occur over the ensuing years. We certainly did not expect that 50 years later our work and its biomedical implications would be the focus of a special commemorative issue of *The American Journal of Psychiatry*, which would later be expanded and republished as a book!

I am deeply gratified, however, that this progression has occurred, and that in 2004 we actually know enough about the relationship between genes and the illnesses that affect the mind and brain to have this topic featured in the world's most widely read psychiatric journal. I am gratified as well that the ramifications are so many and varied. In the 21st century, psychiatrists are being invited to think about animal models of the illnesses they observe daily in human beings and to recognize that these models will aid in the development of new medications to treat mental illnesses. Psychiatrists are being challenged to learn about the new technologies and terminologies—microarrays, haplotype maps, and promotor regions—that have arisen as a consequence of the enormous progress that has occurred in molecular biology. Most important, as this book demonstrates, the tools of molecular biology are now being applied to improve understanding of both normal behavioral variations, and also the mechanisms of a wide variety of complex disorders such as schizophrenia, mood disorders, and substance abuse.

I am confident that during the upcoming years the heritage of the double helix will help psychiatrists, neuroscientists, and behavioral scientists unlock many secrets of the mind and brain. Although challenging because of their genetic complexity, mental illnesses are among the most important diseases to be studied with the tools of molecular biology. Their effects are devastating to both patients and their families. Therefore, I proudly look forward to continuing to both foster and follow the discoveries about their mechanisms and treatment that are certain to occur as a consequence of our modest achievement 50 years ago.

James D. Watson, Ph.D.

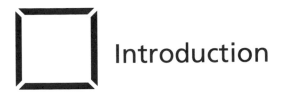

Introduction

From Molecule to Mind: Genetics, Genomics, and Psychiatry

It is likely that in April of 1953 very few psychiatrists took note of a one-page paper in *Nature* written by James Watson and Francis Crick. In fact, it is quite probable that few psychiatrists today have actually read this classic in the history of science, although the enormous attention created by the sequencing of the human genome has certainly placed genetics and genomics on the radar screen for all of us. This book is designed both to commemorate and honor the "double helix discovery" and to prepare psychiatrists for the "genomic era" that will unfold during the 21st century.

We have reprinted the original *Nature* paper here for all to read. We are honored to be able to include some comments by James Watson as well as by Marshall Nirenberg recipient of the 1968 Nobel in Medicine for discovering that RNA is used for protein synthesis. We also have included six highly educational overview chapters by distinguished authors, beginning with an excellent summary and methodological critique by Kenneth Kendler of the various techniques currently being used in psychiatric genetics studies. Thomas Insel and Francis Collins, the Directors of NIMH and the National Human Genome Research Institute, respectively, provide an insightful discussion on the general topic of psychiatry in the genomics era. The subsequent chapters of this book continue the presentation of a variety of genetic perspectives and topics—endophenotypes, animal models, microarrays, and general strategies for identifying the genetic mechanisms of mental illnesses— all written by leaders in the field.

Some of you may be shaking your heads and wondering if all this "technical stuff" really has anything to do with psychiatry, or if it will change your daily practice in any way. Believe me—it will. The question is not a matter of "if" but "when?" So right now is the time to start educating yourself about it, if you haven't already. The genomics era has implications for all of us, whatever our intellectual and philosophical approach to psychiatry and whatever mix of patients we treat.

If the past is any predictor of the future, then I would infer that we cannot come close to imagining how much the genomic revolution will change psychiatry during the next 50 years. As explained by Kathleen Ries Merikangas and Neil Risch, the genetic contributions to major mental illnesses have been well recognized for more than a century. The genetic contributions to other human traits and variations are increasingly being studied and documented, as demonstrated by the article on shyness in this issue. It will take time and a great deal of work, but over the coming decades we are certain to learn much more about the movement from molecules to minds—how our genes contribute to who and what each of us is, and how and why some of us move from the normal continuum into a state of pathology.

As a psychiatrist who has struggled to help people with serious mental illnesses for 30 years, I welcome the era of the genome with great hope. The "genomics era" is about much more than "finding genes." It is about understanding how they get turned on, or turned off. It is about examining the complex interactions between genes and the huge array of nongenetic factors that influence their effects. It is about our capacity as scientists and clinicians to improve diagnosis, treatment, and, ultimately, prevention. The tools described in this issue will gradually and steadily be used to identify new ways to intervene and prevent, or ways to treat more effectively and intelligently.

During the 21st century, a story whose plot we do not yet know will certainly unfold. Whatever its specific content, it will be about how we can move from studying and understanding molecules to studying and understanding the human mind. During this journey from molecule to mind, we will discover many ways to ameliorate and perhaps prevent some of the untold human suffering caused by mental illnesses. Prepare yourselves to understand this journey by reading this book!

Nancy C. Andreasen, M.D., Ph.D.

Molecular Structure of Nucleic Acids

A Structure for Deoxyribose Nucleic Acid

J. D. Watson
F. H. C. Crick

We wish to suggest a structure for the salt of deoxyribose nucleic acid (D.N.A.). This structure has novel features which are of considerable biological interest.

A structure for nucleic acid has already been proposed by Pauling and Corey.[1] They kindly made their manuscript available to us in advance of publication. Their model consists of three intertwined chains, with the phosphates near the fibre axis, and the bases on the outside. In our opinion, this structure is unsatisfactory for two reasons: 1) We believe that the material which gives the X-ray diagrams is the salt, not the free acid. Without the acidic hydrogen atoms it is not clear what forces would hold the structure together, especially as the negatively charged phosphates near the axis will repel each other. 2) Some of the van der Waals distances appear to be too small.

Another three-chain structure has also been suggested by Fraser (in the press). In his model the phosphates are on the outside and the bases on the inside, linked together by hydrogen bonds. This structure as de-

Medical Research Council Unit for the Study of the Molecular Structure of Biological Systems, Cavendish Laboratory, Cambridge. April 2.

Reprinted by permission from *Nature* vol. 171:737–738 (1953). Copyright © 2003 Macmillan Publishers Ltd.

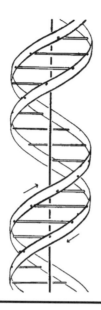

Figure 1.

This figure is purely diagrammatic. The two ribbons symbolize the two phosphate–sugar chains, and the horizontal rods the pairs of bases holding the chains together. The vertical line marks the fibre axis.

scribed is rather ill-defined, and for this reason we shall not comment on it.

We wish to put forward a radically different structure for the salt of deoxyribose nucleic acid. This structure has two helical chains each coiled round the same axis (see diagram). We have made the usual chemical assumptions, namely, that each chain consists of phosphate diester groups joining β-D-deoxyribofuranose residues with 3′,5′ linkages. The two chains (but not their bases) are related by a dyad perpendicular to the fibre axis. Both chains follow right-handed helices, but owing to the dyad the sequences of the atoms in the two chains run in opposite directions. Each chain loosely resembles Furberg's[2] model No. 1; that is, the bases are on the inside of the helix and the phosphates on the outside. The configuration of the sugar and the atoms near it is close to Furberg's 'standard configuration', the sugar being roughly perpendicular to the attached base. There is a residue on each chain every 3.4 A. in the z-direction. We have assumed an angle of 36° between adjacent residues in the same chain, so that the structure repeats after 10 residues on each chain, that is, after 34 A. The distance of a phosphorus atom from the fibre axis is 10 A. As the phosphates are on the outside, cations have easy access to them.

The structure is an open one, and its water content is rather high. At lower water contents we would expect the bases to tilt so that the structure could become more compact.

The novel feature of the structure is the manner in which the two chains are held together by the purine and pyrimidine bases. The planes of the bases are perpendicular to the fibre axis. They are joined together in pairs, a single base from one chain being hydrogen-bonded to a single base from the other chain, so that the two lie side by side with identical z-co-ordinates. One of the pair must be a purine and the other a pyrimidine for bonding to occur. The hydrogen bonds are made as follows: purine position 1 to pyrimidine position 1; purine position 6 to pyrimidine position 6.

If it is assumed that the bases only occur in the structure in the most plausible tautomeric forms (that is, with the keto rather than the enol configurations) it is found that only specific pairs of bases can bond together. These pairs are: adenine (purine) with thymine (pyrimidine), and guanine (purine) with cytosine (pyrimidine).

In other words, if an adenine forms one member of a pair, on either chain, then on these assumptions the other member must be thymine; similarly for guanine and cytosine. The sequence of bases on a single chain does not appear to be restricted in any way. However, if only specific pairs of bases can be formed, it follows that if the sequence of bases on one chain is given, then the sequence on the other chain is automatically determined.

It has been found experimentally[3, 4] that the ratio of the amounts of adenine to thymine, and the ratio of guanine to cytosine, are always very close to unity for deoxyribose nucleic acid.

It is probably impossible to build this structure with a ribose sugar in place of the deoxyribose, as the extra oxygen atom would make too close a van der Waals contact. The previously published X-ray data[5, 6] on deoxyribose nucleic acid are insufficient for a rigorous test of our structure. So far as we can tell, it is roughly compatible with the experimental data, but it must be regarded as unproved until it has been checked against more exact results. Some of these are given in the following communications. We were not aware of the details of the results presented there when we devised our structure, which rests mainly though not entirely on published experimental data and stereochemical arguments.

It has not escaped our notice that the specific pairing we have postulated immediately suggests a possible copying mechanism for the genetic material.

Full details of the structure, including the conditions assumed in building it, together with a set of co-ordinates for the atoms, will be published elsewhere.

We are much indebted to Dr. Jerry Donohue for constant advice and criticism, especially on interatomic distances. We have also been stimulated by a knowledge of the general nature of the unpublished experimental results and ideas of Dr. M.H.F. Wilkins, Dr. R.E. Franklin and their co-workers at King's College, London. One of us (J.D.W.) has been aided by a fellowship from the National Foundation for Infantile Paralysis.

References

1. Pauling L, Corey RB: Nature 1953, 171:346; Proc. U.S. Nat. Acad. Sci. 1953, 39:84
2. Furberg S: Acta Chem. Scand. 1953, 6:634
3. Chargaff E, for references see Zamenhof S, Brawerman G, Chargaff E: Biochim. et Biophys. Acta 1952, 9:402
4. Wyatt GR: J. Gen. Physiol. 1952, 36:201
5. Astbury WT: Symp. Soc. Exp. Biol. 1, Nucleic Acid, 66. Camb. Univ. Press, 1947
6. Wilkins MHF, Randall JT: Biochim. et Biophys. Acta 1953, 10:192

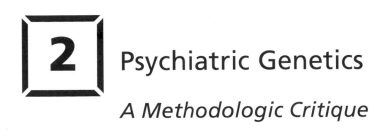

2 | Psychiatric Genetics

A Methodologic Critique

Kenneth S. Kendler, M.D.

Over the last several decades, as the field of psychiatric genetics has grown in size and influence, several distinct paradigms have emerged that approach from different perspectives the goal of understanding the role of genetic factors in the etiology of psychiatric disorders. In this article, I describe these paradigms, review their strengths and weaknesses, summarize scientific progress made in each area, and then explore the conceptual and philosophical issues posed by these paradigms and their interrelationship.

While psychiatric genetic strategies can be useful in clarifying the action of environmental factors, this essay will focus on genetic effects. We will not review problems of statistical power that are critical for all paradigms.

The Four Paradigms—Explication

Paradigm 1—Basic Genetic Epidemiology

As outlined in Table 1, the goal of basic genetic epidemiology is to quantify the degree to which individual differences in risk (more technically "liability") to illness result from familial effects (as assessed by a

Supported in part by NIH grants MH-41953, MH/AA/DA-49492, and DA-11287; the Rachel Brown Banks Endowment Fund; and a Fritz Redlich Fellowship at the Center for Advanced Study in the Behavioral Sciences.

The author thanks Kenneth Schaffner, M.D., Ph.D.; Jonathan Flint, M.D.; and Carol Prescott, Ph.D., for helpful comments on an earlier version.

Table 1. Four major paradigms of psychiatric genetics

Paradigm	Samples studied	Method of inquiry	Scientific goals
1. Basic genetic epidemiology	Family, twin, and adoption studies	Statistical	To quantify the degree of familial aggregation and/or heritability
2. Advanced genetic epidemiology	Family, twin, and adoption studies	Statistical	To explore the nature and mode of action of genetic risk factors
3. Gene finding	High-density families, trios, case-control samples	Statistical	To determine the genomic location and identity of susceptibility genes
4. Molecular genetics	Individuals	Biological	To identify critical DNA variants and trace the biological pathways from DNA to disorder

family study) or genetic factors (as determined by twin or adoption studies). While family, twin, and adoption studies can each be used to address the issues of basic (and advanced) genetic epidemiology, they differ in approach and emphasis. For the sake of simplicity, I focus here on twin studies; twin studies constitute the area of my own expertise, and these studies have seen the greatest recent growth, driven by the widening availability of twin registries[1] and sophisticated analytic tools.[2]

For twin studies, the task of basic genetic epidemiology is to estimate the proportion of liability in a given population due to genetic differences between individuals. This proportion is called heritability. The statistical model that forms the basis of these calculations (the liability-threshold model)[3,4] assumes a sufficiently large number of individual genetic and environmental risk factors of sufficiently small individual effect that the central limit theorem applies—that is, the resulting distribution of liability in the population approximates normality.[5] In this essay, I refer to "genes" identified by genetic epidemiologic methods as genetic risk factors to distinguish them from susceptibility genes, which are identified by paradigms 3 and 4.

Paradigm 2—Advanced Genetic Epidemiology

Given the demonstration of significant heritability, the goal of advanced genetic epidemiology is to explore the nature and mode of action of these genetic risk factors. Potential questions include:[6,7]

1. Are these genetic risk factors specific to a given disorder or shared with other psychiatric or substance use disorders?
2. Do these genetic risk factors affect disease risk similarly in males and females?
3. To what extent are the effects of these genetic risk factors mediated through intermediate phenotypes such as personality or neuropsychological processes?
4. Do these genetic risk factors moderate the effect of environmental risk factors on disease liability (genetic control of sensitivity to the environment)?[8]
5. Do these genetic risk factors affect disease risk through altering the probability of exposure to environmental risk factors (genetic control of exposure to the environment)?[8]
6. Does the action of these risk factors change as a function of the developmental stage of the individual?
7. Do historical experiences moderate the effect of genetic risk factors so that heritability might differ across historical cohorts?
8. For disorders that have multiple stages (e.g., substantial alcohol consumption must proceed from but does not always lead to alcohol dependence), what is the relationship between the genetic risk factors for these various stages?
9. Does the level of heritability for a disorder differ across populations?

In both the basic and advanced genetic epidemiologic research paradigms, genetic risk factors are not directly measured. Rather their existence is inferred—by using well-understood statistical methods—from the patterns of resemblance among particular classes of relatives such as monozygotic versus dizygotic twins or biological parents and their adopted-away offspring.

Paradigm 3—Gene Finding

The goal of gene finding methods is to determine the locations on the genome of genes (or more technically loci) variation, which influences liability to psychiatric disorders. While molecular methods are used for detecting the genetic variants (or "markers") that are critical to these analyses, gene finding methods are statistical in nature. By examining the distribution of genetic markers within families or populations, these methods (linkage and/or association) infer the probability that a locus in the genomic region under investigation contributes to disease liability. A further and more refined goal for paradigm 3 is to clarify the history of the pathogenic variant or variants in the susceptibility gene by determining the background pieces of DNA (termed "haplotypes") on which these variants are found.

Paradigm 4—Molecular Genetics

The goal of the molecular genetic paradigm in psychiatric genetics is to trace the biological mechanisms by which the DNA variant identified with gene finding methods contributes to the disorder itself. The first and most critical goal is to identify the change in gene function and/or expression resulting from the identified DNA variant. The more complex goal involves the use of a wide range of methods (e.g., molecular, pharmacological, imaging, neuropsychological) to trace, at a basic biological level, the etiologic pathway(s) from the DNA variant to the abnormal brain/mind functioning that characterizes the disorder.

The Four Paradigms—Strengths and Limitations

Basic Genetic Epidemiology

Basic genetic epidemiology has the following important strengths:

1. The convincing demonstration of heritability allows for the definitive rejection of the "radical environmentalist" position, which asserts that a clustering of illness within families is ipso facto evidence for the importance of familial-environmental risk factors. For example, it has been argued that the familial clustering of schizophrenia and schizophrenia spectrum traits such as deviant communication patterns indicates that schizophrenia can be "taught" by parents to their children.[9] In the psychological, sociological or epidemiologic literature, papers can still be found that assume that parental smoking is a psychosocial risk factor for smoking[10] or that parent-offspring transmission of romantic relationship style[11] can be assumed to be a result solely of social learning.
2. Basic genetic epidemiologic methods assess the aggregate effects of all genetic risk factors regardless of their location on the genome or their individual effect size. These methods therefore provide an

overall assessment for a given population of the etiologic importance of genetic variation.

3. Positive results from the basic method—the clear demonstration of genetic risk factors—provides a foundation for further work in which the methods of advanced genetic epidemiology are used.

Basic genetic epidemiologic methods have the following critical limitations:

1. The ultimate goal of science is commonly conceived to be the elucidation of causal processes. By this criterion, the basic genetic epidemiologic paradigm is unsatisfactory because it is fundamentally descriptive in nature. While this method quantifies the importance of genetic risk factors, it provides no insight into causal or explanatory pathways.
2. Heritability estimates apply to populations and not to individuals. Indeed, the heritability of a disorder in an individual is undefined.
3. In a given population with a particular set of genes, the heritability of a disorder is not immutable and would change by the introduction of new sources of environmental risk. Thus, the magnitude of heritability is not solely a result of gene action. Rather, it is a ratio of the variance in risk in a population due to genetic differences between individuals and the total variance of risk in that population. There is no a priori reason why the heritability of a disorder should be the same across different human populations or historical periods, which likely contain differences in the distribution of both genetic and environmental risk factors. Therefore, contrary to common usage, "heritability" does *not* designate a characteristic of a disorder or a trait but only of a disorder or trait in a specific population at a specific time.
4. The liability-threshold model that underlies most genetic epidemiologic analyses is biologically nonspecific and quite divorced from actual genetic processes. The assumptions of this model (large number of risk loci with very small individual effects) constitute a biological null hypothesis, which is difficult to reject but provides little insight into underlying biological processes.
5. The relationship between heritability and feasibility of gene finding is strong only at one extreme; if heritability is zero, gene finding methods will not succeed. However, given nonzero heritability estimates, the magnitude of these estimates provides little to no information about the ease of gene finding. This is because heritability estimates assess only aggregate genetic effect and are uninformative

about the distribution of genetic risk across the genome. It can be easy to find genes for traits with low heritability if most of that genetic risk is concentrated in one genomic location and/or the genetic effects are particularly strong only in some families. It can be very difficult to localize genetic risk for a disorder with high heritability if the disorder is influenced slightly by variation at many loci widely spread throughout the genome. For example, while the heritability of breast cancer is modest,[12] researchers have identified two major genes (BRCA1 and BRCA2)[13] in which mutations can occur that are responsible for a large proportion of familial breast cancers.

6. For the estimate of heritability, twin studies rely critically on excess phenotypic resemblance in monozygotic versus dizygotic twins. Nongenetic processes that cause such excess resemblance will bias heritability estimates. While evidence suggests that such biases are probably not large,[6] the observational, nonexperimental nature of genetic epidemiology makes it difficult to rule out such biases definitively.

Advanced Genetic Epidemiology

The most important strength of advanced genetic epidemiologic methods is that they move beyond the descriptive approach of paradigm 1 to an exploration of the action of genetic risk factors. Some of these methods, for example, incorporate environmental risk factors or intermediate phenotypes in the analyses. Most important, many of these methods begin to address questions of causal processes (e.g., questions 3–8 listed earlier).

The major limitations of the advanced genetic epidemiologic methods are extensions of the limitations listed earlier for the basic methods—especially points 2, 3, and 6. While such advanced methods can approach causal issues, they are addressed by tracing processes between latent statistically defined genetic risk factors. For example, the latent genetic risk factors for major depression and schizophrenia may act in part by influencing the personality trait of neuroticism[14,15] and attentional and executive processes,[16,17] respectively. Since neuroticism and attention may be more basic constructs than major depression and schizophrenia, these analyses would constitute a reductive form of explanation—that is explaining a higher-order complex phenomenon as a manifestation of simpler, more basic processes. However, advanced genetic epidemiology offers only partial reductive explanations involving several adjacent levels of a complex causal chain. These causal explanations cannot reach the level of basic genetic/biological processes, such as DNA base-pair variation.[18]

Gene Finding

Gene finding methods have the following critical strengths:

1. While statistical in nature, these methods have underlying assumptions that are firmly based on the well-characterized biological process of meiosis—that is genetic recombination and segregation.
2. The results of gene finding methods are more specific, informative, and falsifiable than those from basic genetic epidemiology. By most criteria, these characteristics mean that the results of gene finding methods would have greater scientific value.[19]
3. Because these methods are based on sound and well-understood genetic principles, positive results for gene finding methods present a natural basis for further work with the molecular genetic paradigm.

Gene finding methods have the following critical limitations:

1. As with heritability calculations, the statistical methods for gene localization do not solely reflect gene action but rather assess the ratio of genetic to total variance in liability. The evidence for linkage in a family would vary as a function of the potency and frequency of the environmental risk factors to which its members were exposed.
2. While gene finding methods detect susceptibility genes over small regions of the genome, there is no guarantee that the actual susceptibility gene itself will be easy to determine. Even with relatively large samples, the size of the "high-risk" region detected by linkage analysis can be quite large, containing dozens to hundreds of possible susceptibility genes.[20] In experimental organisms, examples are now emerging of single "signals," obtained by gene finding methods, that on closer examination, turn out to reflect multiple individual genetic loci.[21,22]
3. While basic genetic epidemiology performs one test to determine the presence of genetic risk factors, gene finding methods have to perform many individual tests to detect susceptibility genes. Because genetic risk factors have been found for nearly all psychiatric and drug abuse disorders examined to date, the hypothesis tested in paradigm 1 (e.g., genetic risk factors exist for disorder X) has a high a priori probability. By contrast, the hypothesis tested in gene finding methods (that a small region of the genome contains a susceptibility gene for disorder X) is much less likely to be true. Statistical theory predicts that positive results from basic genetic epidemiology studies (one test with high a priori probability) will prove much more reliable than positive results from gene finding methods

(many tests with low a priori probabilities). As discussed later in this article, this prediction is well borne out.

Molecular Genetics

Molecular genetics has a single overwhelming strength. That is, its methods raise the possibility of reductive biological explanations that would elucidate the causal chain from molecular variation in DNA to the manifestations of psychiatric disorders. Unlike paradigms 1–3, molecular genetics is not fundamentally statistical in nature but rather reflects the biological reductive model of science that has been frequently successful in biomedicine.

Molecular genetics also has one noteworthy weakness: Many practical problems stand in the way of clarifying what may be the extraordinarily complex biological pathways from DNA variation to psychiatric disorders. The individual genetic variants that cause classic genetic disorders are usually easy to detect because they reflect alterations in coding for key amino acids or the destruction of well-defined regulatory sequences. However, the DNA variants that predispose to complex diseases (including psychiatric disorders) may be more subtle in their action and more difficult to detect. Efforts to understand in basic biological terms even the simplest of behaviors in model organisms have met with substantial difficulties.[23,24] Molecular genetics also needs to be concerned about how disease risk arises from interactions between genetically controlled biological processes and environmentally induced changes in brain function.

However, the power of molecular biology and neuroscience is also increasing rapidly, so there is reason for guarded optimism that if pathogenic DNA variants are found for psychiatric disorders, it will be ultimately possible to use these variants to gain invaluable insights into the etiology of these disorders.

The Four Paradigms—Selective Review of Current Status

In this section my goal is to provide a brief survey of the current status of knowledge in these four paradigm areas so as to inform the following discussion of interrelationships among the paradigms.

Basic Genetic Epidemiology

Familial and more specifically genetic risk factors have been found for every psychiatric and drug use disorder that has been the subject of serious study. For most disorders, evidence for genetic risk factors has by now been replicated by using the same research design (most commonly twin studies), and for some disorders (e.g., schizophrenia and alcoholism), the evidence has been replicated across twin and adoption designs. For several disorders (including alcoholism, drug abuse, and depression), twin studies with broadly comparable results have been conducted by using clinical and epidemiologic methods of ascertainment. With only a few exceptions, the consistency of results across studies has been high, and this consistency has been confirmed by the first series of meta-analyses.[25–28]

As results have accumulated, it has become clear that heritability estimates probably differ meaningfully between disorders, with the highest heritability found for schizophrenia and bipolar illness and the lowest for anxiety disorders. The heritability of alcohol and drug use disorders is at least as high as that found for more traditional psychiatric disorders such as depression and bulimia. Unless there are strong and consistent methodologic biases operating across study designs, this growing body of work indicates that genetic risk factors are of substantial etiologic importance for all major psychiatric and drug use disorders.

Advanced Genetic Epidemiology

A wide variety of work has been produced in recent years with this paradigm. This review focuses on six areas. First, a number of adoption and twin studies have provided evidence for genotype-by-environment interaction. Genetic risk factors may frequently influence liability to psychiatric disorders by moderating the pathogenic effect of environmental risk factors. Second, a number of multivariate analyses have indicated that genetic risk factors are often not specific for individual psychiatric or drug abuse diagnoses but rather influence liability for a range of disorders. Sets of genetic risk factors are unlikely to map cleanly onto the nosologic categories of DSM-IV-TR or ICD-10. Third, a number of classic "environmental" risk factors for psychiatric illness, including stressful life events, social support, and the quality of parenting, are moderately influenced by genetic factors. Genetic risk factors may influence susceptibility to psychiatric disorders in part by altering the probability of exposure to certain environmental stressors. Fourth, sex effects may be as important in psychiatric genetics as they have long proven to be in psychiatric epidemiology. The genetic risk factors for several common psychiatric disorders may not be entirely the same in men and women. Fifth, partially distinct genetic risk factors act at the multiple stages in the development of substance abuse and dependence. The genetic risk factors influencing the probability of misusing a substance are only partly correlated with those factors that affect risk for initiation of substance use. Sixth, key transitional events in human development may moderate the effect of genetic risk factors. For example, the genetic risk factors that predispose to anxiety disorders in pre-pubertal girls may increase the risk for depression after puberty.

Gene Finding

A very large number of candidate gene association studies have been reported for numerous psychiatric and drug abuse disorders. The interpretation of these findings remains problematic. Recent reviews have documented what many suspected—that a substantial proportion of positive results in gene association studies for complex disorders do not survive the test of replication.[29,30] Probably only one association finding (variation in aldehyde dehydrogenase activity and risk for alcoholism in Asian populations) is well understood biologically, has been consistently replicated, and has proven to have a substantial effect on risk. A number of other findings have been replicated more frequently than expected by chance and may reflect true positive findings.

Whole genome linkage scans have been reported for many psychiatric and substance use disorders, including schizophrenia, bipolar disorder, alcoholism, autism, attention deficit hyperactivity disorder, bulimia, panic disorder, nicotine dependence, and major depression. A sufficient number of linkage studies of schizophrenia and bipolar illness have been conducted to show that the rate of replication of positive regions across studies has been low. This pattern contrasts strikingly with the high level of consistency seen in the results of basic genetic epidemiologic studies—for example, the results of twin and family studies of schizophrenia.[31]

Rigorous meta-analyses of linkage studies of psychiatric disorders are beginning to appear. Particularly noteworthy are two recent studies that utilized raw results of genome linkage scans for schizophrenia and bipolar illness.[32,33] The agreement in regions showing linkage was substantially in excess of chance expectations for schizophrenia, but the results were less clear for bipolar illness.

The last year has seen encouraging advances with a positional candidate gene strategy, in which association methods are applied to genomic regions identified through linkage results. Variants in several genes that appear to affect risk for schizophrenia have been found by using these methods, and replications are appearing for some of them.[34] This field is moving quickly and is likely to have changed substantially by the time this article is in print. Increasing efforts have also been made, with some success, to clarify the DNA background (or haplotypes) on which the pathogenic variants in these susceptibility genes occur (e.g., references 35 and 36).

Molecular Genetics

We have, in the last year, seen the first really viable efforts to trace the biological pathways from potential susceptibility genes to psychiatric phenotypes. For example, mice were developed in which neuregulin 1, one of the recently identified potential susceptibility genes for schizophrenia, was knocked out (rendered nonfunctional).[37] These mice demonstrated reduced expression of N-methyl-D-aspartic acid receptors and abnormalities in prepulse inhibition—a neuropsychological feature found to be, on average, impaired in patients with schizophrenia. Efforts have begun to try to define a common pathway for the molecular affects of identified potential susceptibility genes in deficits that might form part of the pathway from susceptibility genes to the clinical phenotype of schizophrenia.[34]

The Four Paradigms—Interrelationships

Within the field of psychiatric genetics, how should these paradigms interrelate? Positive results from paradigm 1 lead directly to questions posed in paradigm 2. To confirm the statistical signals of gene finding studies (paradigm 3), it is natural to study the biological changes produced by these genetic variants (paradigm 4). More problematic is the nature of the relationship between paradigms 1 and 2 (hereafter genetic epidemiology) and paradigms 3 and 4 (hereafter gene identification).

The crux of this problem is the relationship between genetic risk factors as defined by genetic epidemiology and susceptibility genes as defined by gene identification methods. (This issue is similar, but not identical to, a long-standing debate in the philosophy of biology about the relationship between classic or Mendelian genetics and molecular genetics [see chapters 6 and 7 in reference 38].) Our problem is how to answer a deceptively simple question—are genetic risk factors simply the statistical signals of susceptibility genes? This question can be framed in more philosophical language as, Do genetic risk factors reduce to susceptibility genes?

This central question must be evaluated with great care, because it can be addressed on two different levels with divergent answers. On a theoretical level, the results of twin and adoption studies, if properly conducted, should reflect the distal effects of genetic variation coded in DNA. (No one actively working in psychiatric genetics argues seriously that heritability as assessed in twin or adoption studies emerges from a vitalistic force, although this was advocated in the past in both biological and philosophical circles.) At this theoretical level, therefore, the answer to this question is clear—genetic risk factors are nothing more than signals of susceptibility genes.

However, at a practical level, the answer is more murky in at least two important ways. First, it can be genuinely debated whether it will ever be possible, regardless of technological advances, to trace in a clear and unambiguous fashion a complete set of causal links from DNA base-pair variation to a complex biobehavioral phenomenon such as schizophrenia or major depression. Advocates of these sorts of reductive models argue correctly that the power of emerging technologies to address seemingly intractable scientific questions has more often been under- than overestimated. Furthermore, new analytic methods (such as network theory,[39] which could replace unrealistically simplistic linear causal models) may provide an important impetus for further advances. However, the problems of psychiatric illness, involving some of the most complex conceivable questions, including questions of consciousness, self-concept, and reality testing, may involve emergent properties that are not predictable from basic biological phenomena such as DNA variation.

Second, if genetic risk factors are merely manifestations of susceptibility genes, we should be able to use paradigm 3 to confirm the results of paradigm 1. If there is a dispute about whether a twin or adoption study was correct in its conclusion that disorder X is heritable, then we should be able to evaluate these results by linkage and/or association studies. However, while this idea may seem sensible, it is, in practical terms, wrong. If a twin study of disorder X indicated a heritability of 40% and a well-conducted genome scan showed no regions of significant linkage, it would not be sound to argue, on the basis of the linkage result, that the twin study was in error.

The reason for this apparently paradoxical situation is largely the blunt power of gene identification methods combined with the possibility that genetic risk factors may reflect the combined signal of many susceptibility genes of small individual effect. With an infinite sample size, genotyping methods without error, and yet-to-be-designed statistical tools, it might be theoretically possible for gene identification methods to uncover all of the susceptibility genes that form the biological basis for genetic risk factors and to clarify how they combine and interact to produce a specific level of disease liability. Whether such findings will ever be possible is open to debate. If they will be, we are currently a very long way from that goal.

The practical difficulty of moving from paradigms 1 and 2 to paradigms 3 and 4 leaves a gap in the conceptual framework of psychiatric genetics. It is not yet clear whether we can easily get from genetic risk factors to susceptibility genes. Therefore, genetic epidemiologic and gene identification paradigms do not currently relate to one another as do many paradigms in the physical sciences, in which results at a more abstract level can be clearly reduced to more basic methods and definitively confirmed or refuted by the application of these more basic methods.

Competing Paradigms

Some historical periods in science are marked by competing paradigms.[40] Such a historical/sociological perspective can be usefully applied to the field of psychiatric genetics, where the two broad camps that have adopted genetic epidemiology or gene identification methods as their main paradigm struggle with each other to attract resources and students. Members of these two groups often attend different scientific meetings. Stereotypes have developed among genetic epidemiologists, who characterize molecular geneticists as "gene jocks." Gene finders in turn describe genetic epidemiologists as "just interested in statistics—not in real genes." Over recent years, gene identification methods have gained in prominence, partly at the expense of genetic epidemiologic approaches.

Competition between scientific paradigms most commonly results in one of two outcomes: replacement or integration. In replacement, one paradigm loses, disappearing from the scientific scene. This was the resolution of the competition between the Ptolemaic and Copernican models for planetary motion. In integration, the two paradigms are incorporated into a unified approach. For example, the older paradigm might serve as a useful approximation for the newer paradigm in a limited set of circumstances. While the interpretation is not without controversy (see references 40 and 41), many would see the retention of Newtonian mechanics after the introduction of the theory of relativity (because, with commonly encountered speeds and masses, the two systems produce indistinguishable predictions) as an example of integration of scientific paradigms.

Which of these models best applies to the competing paradigms within psychiatric genetics? While the future is uncertain, a time may come when it is easy and cheap to sequence individual genomes and sufficient statistical tools have been developed that gene identification methods will completely replace genetic epidemiology. Instead of having to infer genetic risk factors from patterns of resemblance across relatives, as is now done in genetic epidemiologic paradigms, it may be possible to measure directly all relevant variants within susceptibility genes and to combine this information with relevant environmental exposures to determine individual liability. These developments would allow a great increase in statistical power because genetic risk could be determined directly and would not need to be inferred by the risk of illness in relatives.

However, if they are ever achievable, such capabilities will not be available for a substantial period of time. Therefore, the field of psychiatric genetics would be better served currently by working toward a model of integration. Such a model would require an appreciation of the complementary sources of information obtained by genetic epidemiologic and gene identification approaches. The major advantage of genetic epidemiologic methods is that they permit us to assess the magnitude of total genetic influences and then explore how those influences act and interact with various aspects of the internal and external environment. However, most of these questions can also be addressed by using gene identification methods, but only at the level of specific genes or genomic regions. Two examples will illustrate this development. Advanced genetic epidemiology has suggested that the genetic risk factors for the personality trait of neuroticism may be correlated but not identical in men and women.[14,42] A linkage study of neuroticism has recently suggested specific genomic locations for these genes that have different effects in the two sexes.[43] A prior twin study suggested that genetic risk factors for major depression in part acted through increasing sensitivity to the depressogenic effects of stressful life events.[44] A recent association study has suggested that having a variant in the serotonin transporter gene increases an individual's risk for developing depression after exposure to high levels of stress.[45] These two kinds of knowledge (at the aggregate level for all genetic risk factors and at the level of specific susceptibility genes) are by their nature complementary.

However, there are important questions asked of psychiatric genetics that can be well answered only at the level of aggregate risk. Examples of scenarios involving such questions would include:

1. A large private foundation wants to invest considerable research funds in investigating the etiology of disorder X. In determining how to divide these funds between strategies emphasizing genetic versus environmental risk factors, the foundation representatives turn to psychiatric genetics and ask, "Overall, how important are genetic versus environmental risk factors for disorder X?"

2. A committee for DSM-V is having a hard time determining whether syndromes A and B should be placed in the same or different diagnostic categories. They plan to collect data on several diagnostic validators, such as response to treatment and course. However, given prior evidence that both syndromes are heritable, they are particularly hopeful that genetic studies will provide definitive information to clarify how closely related the genetic risk factors are for these two disorders.

3. A state legislature is considering a large program to reduce youths' access to alcohol, with the hope that the program will reduce future rates of alcoholism. They know that early onset of alcohol use is associated with later alcoholism but turn to psychiatric genetics to help them evaluate whether that link is causal. Does early onset of alcohol use actually cause future alcoholism, or is the association between early onset of alcohol use and later alcoholism a result of their both being manifestations of an underlying (partly genetic) liability to deviancy?

4. A research team is funded to conduct a large controlled trial of antipsychotic agents in individuals with schizotypal personality disorder. To increase their chances of obtaining positive results, they turn to psychiatric genetics to obtain a definition of this disorder that maximizes its genetic relationship to schizophrenia.

In each of these scenarios, the question cannot be currently answered by using gene identification methods. It requires the ability to assess total genetic risk—currently only possible with genetic epidemiologic methods.

Psychiatric Genetics and Reductive Models for Psychopathology

This review of the relative merits of genetic epidemiologic and gene identification approaches to psychiatric genetics can be productively viewed as part of a broader discussion about the relative value of "hard" reductive models in psychiatry versus "explanatory pluralism."[46] With the remarkable advances in neuroscience and molecular biology, an increasingly common view within psychiatry, and especially biological psychiatry, is that the only valid etiologic models for psychiatric disorders are in basic biological or molecular terms. By contrast, advocates of explanatory pluralism would argue that our ignorance about the underlying causes of psychiatric illness is so profound that we are not in a position to be so selective about the origins of our knowledge. We should not reject, they would argue, partial etiologic explanations, even when they are expressed in nonbiological terms. They would see this kind of patchy reduction to be a much more realistic goal than a complete top-to-bottom hard reductive model.[47]

(Advocates of explanatory pluralism are also often skeptical of the claims of hard reductive models that typically assume clear one-to-one relationships between basic biological processes—such as DNA variants in a susceptibility gene—and psychiatric disorders. They would argue that the intervening processes are of such complexity that "many-to-many" relationships are much more likely, because many different susceptibility genes would predispose to one disorder, and variants in one susceptibility gene could, depending on other genes or environmental exposure, predispose to different disorders.)

The question of the relationship between "hard reduction" and explanatory pluralism can be best illustrated by a thought experiment. Imagine there were 15 levels of the mind/brain system separating DNA variants and the clinical diagnosis of major depression. (These levels would include processes best conceptualized within a biological framework, such as intracellular signal pathways, cellular organization, local synaptic connections, and neuroanatomical pathways, as well as constructs best understood within a psychological framework, including attachment history, self-esteem, and personality.) Gene identification methods have predominantly focused on trying to directly connect level 1 (DNA variation) to level 15 (major depression).

While complex genetic epidemiology has begun to evaluate reductive models, they differ from those explored by gene identification methods. Consider the evidence that genetic risk factors for the personality trait of neuroticism are closely related to the genetic risk factors for major depression.[14] In our thought experiment, this study might be seen as having established a link between level 12 (personality) and level 15 (major depression). Is this study a useful contribution to the psychiatric genetics literature?

Advocates of hard reductive models would argue "no," probably claiming that all this research does is relate a fuzzy psychiatric disorder to an equally fuzzy psychological construct. For them, a reductive model has to go all the way down to basic biological processes to be valid and useful. By contrast, advocates of explanatory pluralism would argue that this study has produced a useful insight, by making an etiologic connection between two different scientific constructs (personality and psychopathology) at somewhat different levels of abstraction, each having its own literature and set of associated insights.

Conclusion

Psychiatric genetics currently employs a range of research paradigms that can be usefully organized into four groups: basic genetic epidemiology, advanced genetic epidemiology, gene finding methods, and molecular genetics. In this article, I explored the methods employed and the questions asked in each of these paradigms and then briefly reviewed the current status of work in each area. Due to both practical research limitations and the potential theoretical properties of complex systems, a substantial conceptual discontinuity divides the field. It is not clear how easy it will be to get from genetic risk factors, as determined by genetic epidemiologic methods, to susceptibility genes, as determined by molecular genetics.

While genetic epidemiology may eventually be replaced by gene identification methods, this development is sufficiently far in the future that the field of psychiatric genetics will benefit from attempts to integrate these various paradigms, which will require an appreciation of their complementary strengths and limitations. The optimal framework within which to pursue this integration is one of explanatory pluralism, which requires the realization that a restriction to hard reductionist models is counterproductive, given the current immature status of the science. Partial or patchy reductions—for which genetic epidemiologic models are particularly well suited—have an important role to play in future advances in the field.

References

1. Busjahn A: Twin registers across the globe: what's out there in 2002? (editorial). Twin Res 2002; 5:v–vi
2. Neale MC, Boker SM, Xie G, Maes HH: Mx: Statistical Modeling, 5th ed. Richmond, Va, Medical College of Virginia of Virginia Commonwealth University, Department of Psychiatry, 1999
3. Fisher RA: On the correlation between relatives on the supposition of Mendelian inheritance. Trans R Soc Edinburgh 1918; 52:399–433
4. Falconer DS: The inheritance of liability to certain diseases, estimated from the incidence among relatives. Ann Hum Genet 1965; 29:51–76
5. Kendler KS, Kidd KK: Recurrence risks in an oligogenic threshold model: the effect of alterations in allele frequency. Ann Hum Genet 1986; 50(part 1):83–91
6. Kendler KS: Twin studies of psychiatric illness: current status and future directions. Arch Gen Psychiatry 1993; 50:905–915
7. Kendler KS: Twin studies of psychiatric illness: an update. Arch Gen Psychiatry 2001; 58:1005–1014

8. Kendler KS, Eaves LJ: Models for the joint effect of genotype and environment on liability to psychiatric illness. Am J Psychiatry 1986; 143:279–289

9. Lidz T, Fleck S, Cornelison AR: Schizophrenia and the Family. New York, International Universities Press, 1965

10. Tyas SL, Pederson LL: Psychosocial factors related to adolescent smoking: a critical review of the literature. Tob Control 1998; 7:409–420

11. Conger RD, Cui M, Bryant CM, Elder GH Jr: Competence in early adult romantic relationships: a developmental perspective on family influences. J Pers Soc Psychol 2000; 79:224–237

12. Lichtenstein P, Holm NV, Verkasalo PK, Iliadou A, Kaprio J, Koskenvuo M, Pukkala E, Skytthe A, Hemminki K: Environmental and heritable factors in the causation of cancer—analyses of cohorts of twins from Sweden, Denmark, and Finland. N Engl J Med 2000; 343:78–85

13. Moynahan ME: The cancer connection: BRCA1 and BRCA2 tumor suppression in mice and humans. Oncogene 2002; 21:8994–9007

14. Fanous A, Gardner CO, Prescott CA, Cancro R, Kendler KS: Neuroticism, major depression and gender: a population-based twin study. Psychol Med 2002; 32:719–728

15. Kendler KS, Gardner CO, Prescott CA: Toward a comprehensive developmental model for major depression in women. Am J Psychiatry 2002; 159:1133–1145

16. Cannon TD, Huttunen MO, Lonnqvist J, Tuulio-Henriksson A, Pirkola T, Glahn D, Finkelstein J, Hietanen M, Kaprio J, Koskenvuo M: The inheritance of neuropsychological dysfunction in twins discordant for schizophrenia. Am J Hum Genet 2000; 67:369–382

17. Goldberg TE, Torrey EF, Gold JM, Bigelow LB, Ragland RD, Taylor E, Weinberger DR: Genetic risk of neuropsychological impairment in schizophrenia: a study of monozygotic twins discordant and concordant for the disorder. Schizophr Res 1995; 17:77–84

18. Sarkar S: Genetics and Reductionism. New York, Cambridge University Press, 1998

19. Chalmers AF: What Is This Thing Called Science? An Assessment of the Nature and Status of Science and Its Methods, 3rd ed. Indianapolis, Hackett, 1999

20. Roberts SB, MacLean CJ, Neale MC, Eaves LJ, Kendler KS: Replication of linkage studies of complex traits: an examination of the variation in location estimates. Am J Hum Genet 1999; 65:876–884

21. Legare ME, Bartlett FS II, Frankel WN: A major effect QTL determined by multiple genes in epileptic EL mice. Genome Res 2000; 10:42–48

22. Talbot CJ, Radcliffe RA, Fullerton J, Hitzemann R, Wehner JM, Flint J: Fine scale mapping of a genetic locus for conditioned fear. Mamm Genome 2003; 14:223–230

23. Schaffner KF: Genes, behavior, and developmental emergentism: one process, indivisible? Philos Sci 1998; 65:209–252

24. de Bono M, Tobin DM, Davis MW, Avery L, Bargmann CI: Social feeding in Caenorhabditis elegans is induced by neurons that detect aversive stimuli. Nature 2002; 419:899–903

25. Kendler KS, Gardner CO Jr: The risk for psychiatric disorders in relatives of schizophrenic and control probands: a comparison of three independent studies. Psychol Med 1997; 27:411–419

26. Sullivan PF, Neale MC, Kendler KS: Genetic epidemiology of major depression: review and meta-analysis. Am J Psychiatry 2000; 157:1552–1562

27. Li MD, Cheng R, Ma JZ, Swan GE: A meta-analysis of estimated genetic and environmental effects on smoking behavior in male and female adult twins. Addiction 2003; 98:23–31

28. Sullivan PF, Kendler KS, Neale JM: Schizophrenia as a complex trait: evidence from a meta-analysis of twin studies. Arch Gen Psychiatry 2003; 60:1187–1192

29. Lohmueller KE, Pearce CL, Pike M, Lander ES, Hirschhorn JN: Meta-analysis of genetic association studies supports a contribution of common variants to susceptibility to common disease. Nat Genet 2003; 33:177–182

30. Ioannidis JP, Trikalinos TA, Ntzani EE, Contopoulos-Ioannidis DG: Genetic associations in large versus small studies: an empirical assessment. Lancet 2003; 361:567–571

31. Riley BP, Kendler KS: Schizophrenia: genetic epidemiology, in Kaplan and Sadock's Comprehensive Textbook of Psychiatry, 8th Edition. Edited by Sadock BJ, Sadock VA. Philadelphia, Lippincott, Williams and Wilkins (in press)

32. Lewis CM, Levinson DF, Wise LH, DeLisi L, Straub RE, Hovatta I, Williams NM, Schwab SG, Pulver AE, Faraone S, Brzustowicz LM, Kaufmann CA, Garver DL, Gurling HM, Lindholm E, Coon H, Moises HW, Byerley W, Shaw SH, Mesen A, Sherrington R, O'Neill FA, Walsh D, Kendler KS, Ekelund J, Paunio T, Lonnqvist J, Peltonen L, O'Donovan MC, Owen MJ, Wildenauer DB, Maier W, Nestadt G, Blouin JL, Antonarakis SE, Mowry BJ, Silverman JM, Crowe RR, Cloninger CR, Tsuang MT, Malaspina D, Harkavy-Friedman JM, Svrakic DM, Bassett AS, Holcomb J, Kalsi G, McQuillin A, Brynjolfsson J, Sigmundsson T, Petursson H, Jazin E, Zoega T, Helgason T: Genome scan meta-analysis of schizophrenia and bipolar disorder, part II. Am J Hum Genet 2003; 73:34–48

33. Segurado R, Detera-Wadleigh SD, Levinson DF, Lewis CM, Gill M, Nurnberger JI Jr, Craddock N, DePaulo JR, Baron M, Gershon ES, Ekholm J, Cichon S, Turecki G, Claes S, Kelsoe JR, Schofield PR, Badenhop RF, Morissette J, Coon H, Blackwood D, McInnes LA, Foroud T, Edenberg HJ, Reich T, Rice JP, Goate A, McInnis MG, McMahon FJ, Badner JA, Goldin LR, Bennett P, Willour VL, Zandi PP, Liu J, Gilliam C, Juo SH, Berrettini WH, Yoshikawa T, Peltonen L, Lonnqvist J, Nothen MM, Schumacher J, Windemuth C, Rietschel M, Propping P, Maier W, Alda M, Grof P, Rouleau GA, Del-Favero J, Van Broeckhoven C, Mendlewicz J, Adolfsson R, Spence MA, Luebbert H, Adams LJ, Donald JA, Mitchell PB, Barden N,

Shink E, Byerley W, Muir W, Visscher PM, Macgregor S, Gurling H, Kalsi G, McQuillin A, Escamilla MA, Reus VI, Leon P, Freimer NB, Ewald H, Kruse TA, Mors O, Radhakrishna U, Blouin JL, Antonarakis SE, Akarsu N: Genome scan meta-analysis of schizophrenia and bipolar disorder, part III: bipolar disorder. Am J Hum Genet 2003; 73:49–62

34. Harrison PJ, Owen MJ: Genes for schizophrenia? recent findings and their pathophysiological implications. Lancet 2003; 361:417–419

35. Stefansson H, Sarginson J, Kong A, Yates P, Steinthorsdottir V, Gudfinnsson E, Gunnarsdottir S, Walker N, Petursson H, Crombie C, Ingason A, Gulcher JR, Stefansson K, St Clair D: Association of neuregulin 1 with schizophrenia confirmed in a Scottish population. Am J Hum Genet 2003; 72:83–87

36. van den Oord EJ, Sullivan PF, Jiang Y, Walsh D, O'Neill FA, Kendler KS, Riley BP: Identification of a high-risk haplotype for the dystrobrevin binding protein 1 (DTNBP1) gene in the Irish study of high-density schizophrenia families. Mol Psychiatry 2003; 8:499–510

37. Stefansson H, Sigurdsson E, Steinthorsdottir V, Bjornsdottir S, Sigmundsson T, Ghosh S, Brynjolfsson J, Gunnarsdottir S, Ivarsson O, Chou TT, Hjaltason O, Birgisdottir B, Jonsson H, Gudnadottir VG, Gudmundsdottir E, Bjornsson A, Ingvarsson B, Ingason A, Sigfusson S, Hardardottir H, Harvey RP, Lai D, Zhou M, Brunner D, Mutel V, Gonzalo A, Lemke G, Sainz J, Johannesson G, Andresson T, Gudbjartsson D, Manolescu A, Frigge ML, Gurney ME, Kong A, Gulcher JR, Petursson H, Stefansson K: Neuregulin 1 and susceptibility to schizophrenia. Am J Hum Genet 2002; 71:877–892

38. Sterelny K, Griffiths PE: Sex and Death: An Introduction to Philosophy of Biology. Chicago, University of Chicago Press, 1999

39. Jeong H, Tombor B, Albert R, Oltvai ZN, Barabasi AL: The large-scale organization of metabolic networks. Nature 2000; 407:651–654

40. Kuhn TS: The Structure of Scientific Revolutions, 3rd ed. Chicago, University of Chicago Press, 1996

41. Shaffner KF: Discovery and Explanation in Biology and Medicine. Chicago, University of Chicago Press, 1993

42. Eaves LJ, Heath AC, Neale JM, Hewitt JK, Martin NG: Sex differences and non-additivity in the effects of genes on personality. Twin Res 1998; 1:131–137

43. Fullerton J, Cubin M, Tiwari H, Wang C, Bomhra A, Davidson S, Miller S, Fairburn C, Goodwin G, Neale MC, Fiddy S, Mott R, Allison DB, Flint J: Linkage analysis of extremely discordant and concordant sibling pairs identifies quantitative-trait loci that influence variation in the human personality trait neuroticism. Am J Hum Genet 2003; 72:879–890

44. Kendler KS, Kessler RC, Walters EE, MacLean C, Neale MC, Heath AC, Eaves LJ: Stressful life events, genetic liability, and onset of an episode of major depression in women. Am J Psychiatry 1995; 152:833–842

45. Caspi A, Sugden K, Moffitt TE, Taylor A, Craig IW, Harrington H, McClay J, Mill J, Martin J, Braithwaite A, Poulton R: Influence of life stress on depression: moderation by a polymorphism in the 5-HTT gene. Science 2003; 301:386–389

46. Zachar P: Psychological Concepts and Biological Psychiatry: A Philosophical Analysis. Amsterdam, Benjamins, 2000

47. Schaffner KF: Psychiatry and molecular biology: reductionistic approaches to schizophrenia, in Philosophical Perspectives on Psychiatric Diagnostic Classification. Edited by Sadler JZ, Wiggins OP, Schwartz MA. Baltimore, Johns Hopkins University Press, 1994, pp 279–294

3 | Psychiatry in the Genomics Era

Thomas R. Insel, M.D.
Francis S. Collins, M.D., Ph.D.

> We wish to suggest a structure for the salt of deoxyribose nucleic acid (D.N.A.). This structure has novel features which are of considerable biological interest.
>
> *J.D. Watson & F.H.C. Crick*

It has now been 50 years since Watson and Crick's landmark paper on the double helical structure of DNA was published in *Nature* (see Chapter 1).[1] This 1-page paper with a single simple figure and six references sparked a revolution in the life sciences that continued through the latter half of the 20th century, yielding the powerful tools of modern molecular biology, the biotechnology revolution, and, in the past 2 years, the sequencing of the human genome. It is probably a safe bet that, until recently, most readers of *The American Journal of Psychiatry* would have considered this revolution more relevant to their stock portfolios than their clinical practices. As we look beyond the 50th anniversary of the Watson and Crick publication, it is timely to ask whether genomics will become relevant to the practice of psychiatry, and, if so, what the timetable will be. In this commentary we argue that genomics may soon become an important aspect of psychiatry, and we consider what genomics can and cannot do for mental disorders.

Let's start with a few definitions. A gene is simply a sequence of DNA that provides a critical code for messenger RNA, which in turn is translated into protein. How is genomics different from genetics? Genomics and genetics both study the transmission of traits across generations (an interest of Darwin and Freud as well as Mendel). Genetics is the study of single genes and their effects. Genomics is the more ambitious study of all the genes in the genome, including their function, their interaction, and their role in a variety of common disorders that are not due to single genes.[2] Advanced draft descriptions of the human genome have now been published,[3, 4] and the complete sequence is soon expected in public databases. The number of genes is around 30,000, with these genes spaced unevenly across the 2.9 gigabases of DNA that constitute the human genome.

While we note a growing tendency to refer to this period following the sequencing effort as the post-genomic era, we want to emphasize that, from a discovery perspective, we are just entering the genomic era. Certainly, there are many mysteries still to be explained. For instance, less than 2% of the DNA in the genome codes for proteins. The >98% that remains consists of vast repetitive stretches of DNA and other sequences that may have regulatory effects or may be a nonfunctional residual of evolution. While this >98% of the genome has been frequently disregarded as "junk DNA," it almost certainly has important functions still to be discovered. As evidence, a recent comparison of the human and mouse genomes[5] revealed that the protein-coding regions account for less than half of the DNA that has been strongly conserved over the 70 million years since humans and rodents diverged. The conservation of millions of base pairs of DNA that do not code for protein suggests that these regions might be functional. It is certain that some of these conserved segments will be found to be involved in regulating gene expression by serving as target sites for protein factors that regulate transcription. Others may act by producing small RNA fragments that interfere with gene expression or may confer other biological functions not yet understood.

The arrangement of genes across the genome is strikingly uneven. Some chromosomes (17, 19, and 22) are gene dense and some (13, 18, and 21) are sufficiently gene poor that trisomy (having a third copy) is nonlethal. We do not understand the importance, if any, of this variation in gene density across chromosomes, although it may have something to do with position in the interphase nucleus. The number of genes is itself a mystery, with humans having essentially the same number as mice (27,000–30,500),[5] less than twice the number of the nematode *C. elegans* (approx. 19,700)[6] and slightly more than twice the number of the fly *Drosophila* (approx. 13,600).[7] But the relatively low number of genes may be misleading, since the original dogma that each gene specifies only a single protein has now been supplanted by the observation that single genes routinely make multiple proteins through the mechanism of alternative splicing.[8] By alternative arrangements of RNA following transcription of the DNA, 30,000 genes can code for 100,000 proteins. Adding posttranslational modifications (i.e., changes to the protein following translation from RNA) like proteolysis, phosphorylation, and glycosylation may ultimately yield as many as 1,000,000 different human proteins.

Single-Gene Disorders

For nearly 100 years, inherited factors have been recognized in certain families with a Mendelian pattern of transmission. These genetic diseases fall into dominant, recessive, and X-linked modes of inheritance, but all share transmission via a single gene. The online index of the Mendelian Inheritance in Man (OMIM) currently lists mutations in over 1,200 genes that cause single-gene disorders.[9] Most of these diseases are uncommon, and many do not have major psychiatric manifestations, but they collectively have taught us three lessons that are important insights for the role of genomics in psychiatry. First, there is genetic heterogeneity: the same syndrome can result from several different mutations in the same gene or even mutations in different genes. As many as 180 different mutations of the vasopressin (V2) receptor gene have been reported to cause nephrogenic diabetes insipidus,[10] and familial early onset Alzheimer's disease can arise from mutations in the β-amyloid precursor protein, presenilin-1, or presenilin-2.[11, 12] Conversely, there is variable penetrance: the same mutation in the same gene can result in highly variable phenotypic results. For instance, the gene mutation that results in neurofibromatosis type 1 (von Recklinghausen's disease) can manifest as neurofibromas, malignant peripheral nerve sheath tumors, and bone lesions, but the same exact mutation in blood relatives can manifest as a subclinical phenotype with only a few axillary freckles or café-au-lait spots.[13] The extent of pathology, the location of pathology, or the age of onset can be influenced by modifier genes, by environmental factors, or by poorly understood effects that contribute to differences in severity. Finally, a more practical (but less permanent) observation: the discovery of genes for many of these disorders, such as cystic fibrosis or Huntington's chorea, have thus far proven highly informative for investigating the biology of these illnesses but have not yet altered the treatment in any major way. This is an important theoretical as well as practical point. Single-gene diseases are "simple" in terms of the location of the genetic lesion, but they rarely have "simple" or unitary consequences. For instance, a mutation may not only reduce function, it may cause a gain of function of the protein product (as in Huntington's disease, where an abnormal and apparently toxic protein is produced). Moreover, alterations in the function of a single gene almost always exert their effects within a complex cascade of intracellular events (the protein product of the gene mutation seen in neurofibromatosis type 1, for instance, is a negative regulator of *Ras*, an intracellular messenger critical for many kinds of signaling). Successful treatment approaches may therefore ultimately target a downstream mediator (which may be more accessible for drug treatment) and not the abnormal protein product of the gene with the mutation. The point then is that the discovery of a mutation provides an important starting point for understanding the pathophysiology of the disease. Treatment development requires intensive study of these molecular pathways in cultured cells and whole animals to identify the best target for preventing pathology.

Genomics and Psychiatry

We suspect that more than 99% of what has been written about genes and the brain has focused on less than 1% of the genome (about 300 genes). Based on research in the mouse brain, at least 55% of the genes (i.e., roughly 16,500 genes) are expressed in the brain.[14] Thus, we have a treasure trove of new genes to explore, including many that may prove more important than the few neurotransmitters and intracellular signaling molecules that have been studied so intensively these past 50 years.

Although these new genes will teach us much about how the brain develops and functions, we are not likely to find many single-gene Mendelian disorders in psychiatry. Even in autism, which has the highest heritability of any psychiatric disorder, as many as 10 genes have been suggested on the basis of modeling the inheritance pattern.[15] Rather than looking for rare mutations in genes with big effects, complex genetic disorders involve relatively common variations in multiple genes, each of which has a weak effect. In mental disorders, we are therefore looking at multiple factors that cumulatively make an individual susceptible or vulnerable. Moreover, unlike other complex genetic disorders such as hypertension or diabetes, mental disorders have a complex phenotype for which reliable quantitative traits like blood pressure or blood glucose have been difficult to identify and validate. This shortcoming may be partly overcome with the identification of endophenotypes, such as eye tracking, sensorimotor gating, or measures of working memory in schizophrenia, which yield stable quantitative traits more reliable than clinical state for characterizing the transmission of mental disorders.[16]

Finding genetic factors in mental disorders, whether via linkage or association studies, has proven expensive and, until recently, frustrating. In the past year, several promising candidates have emerged as vulnerability genes for schizophrenia, including neuregulin-1, catechol O-methyltransferase, dysbindin, and G72.[17-22] There are promising leads in autism, depression, bipolar disorder, and panic disorder as well.[23] Anyone who follows psychiatric genetics has learned to be careful with new reports of genes for mental disorders, since the history of this field is mired in nonreplications and disappointments. We empathize with healthy skepticism, but we caution against unhealthy cynicism. With the evidence of heritability in all of these disorders, there is no question that susceptibility genes for all of these disorders will ultimately be found. In fact, with the recent initiation of an international project to determine a haplotype map of the entire human genome (which will map variation in large stretches of DNA), the era of whole genome association studies is likely to be only a few years away. Such studies are expected to have much greater power than the family-based linkage studies that have until now been the dominant approach to searching for genetic factors in psychiatric disorders.

As with Mendelian disorders, the hope is that these vulnerability genes will provide a starting point for defining the biology of these disorders. We have seen this unfold with hypertension. The discovery of linkage to a novel gene has led to the elaboration of an entire pathway related to hypertension with a new, exquisite understanding of how altered signaling in the kidney contributes to this syndrome.[24] Clearly, we need such an anchor to inform the molecular exploration of mental disorders. The promise here is even greater, as genetic variation could be used to redefine the disorders, replacing the current diagnostic system, which has no evident biological basis. In this regard, it is worth noting that the syndromes defined by genotype may have much different boundaries than what we have tried to craft with diagnostic manuals based on presenting symptoms. It is also possible that some genotypes will link to a much broader phenotype than what we have identified diagnostically. For instance, a susceptibility gene for all of the common forms of stroke has been reported on 5q12, suggesting that diverse forms of cerebrovascular disease may paradoxically share a common genetic basis.[25] Similarly, we may discover that some of the genes for vulnerability to anorexia nervosa are shared by OCD and depression, with the genotype linked not to a specific disorder but to a perfectionistic, risk-aversive personality style that confers vulnerability to many syndromes.

Although each gene may have weak effects, combining several susceptibility alleles may increase the predictive power. Note, however, that we are talking about predicting susceptibility to mental disorders. Even more than in many other disorders, we expect that the environment will have a powerful effect on the development of mental disorders. A particularly instructive example of this interaction was recently demonstrated for the monoamine oxidase (MAO)-A gene. Children who have been mistreated are at greater risk for violent antisocial behavior. Caspi et al.[26] reported that a genetic variant of the MAO-A gene that increases MAO-A enzyme activity is associated with reduced violent antisocial behavior in male subjects who had been mistreated, but no effect is seen in a nonselected population. The role of vulnerability genes for mental disorders, as with genes for lung cancer or alcoholism, may be to influence the response to environmental factors, including prenatal events. Conversely, we may find genes for resilience or resistance that may have a greater effect than those for vulnerability.

Conclusion

Will genomics change the way we treat psychiatric patients? Almost certainly. It is important to recognize that even a gene with a weak effect may provide a pathway toward new, targeted therapies for schizophrenia or autism, even if the actual targets are downstream from the original gene of interest. This will require considerable research using cell lines and animal models. Equally important, in the very near future we can expect the development of pharmacogenomics, with genetic tests that predict pharmacological treatment response or vulnerability to a particular adverse effect. Such tests could alter psychopharmacology to make drug choice more selective and safer. Indeed, one of the most important consequences of genomics will be to individualize treatment by allowing a clinician to tailor therapy on the basis of the unique genotype of each patient rather than the mean responses of groups of unrelated patients.

Finally, it is important to remember that genomics is a field that is still in its infancy. Having the sequence of the human genome is an important first step, but it is just a beginning. In many ways, it is like having the white pages of the phone directory with all of the numbers and addresses. The white pages are helpful if you know who you are looking for, but useless when something goes wrong and you don't know whom to call. Genomic medicine needs the yellow pages, with the list of all of the mechanics, plumbers, and electricians who can be summoned to fix an abnormal prefrontal cortex or a failing hippocampus.

Writing the yellow pages requires an understanding of the function and the interaction of all of the genes in the genome, which may require another 50 years of research. The promise is huge—for psychiatry as much as the rest of medicine. Watson and Crick[1] ended their paper with the prophetic and understated observation, "It has not escaped our notice that the specific pairing we have postulated immediately suggests a possible copying mechanism for the genetic material." It should not escape our notice now, 50 years later, that we have an opportunity to revolutionize the diagnosis and treatment of mental disorders during this genomic era. Students of the history of psychiatry looking back from the Watson and Crick centennial in 2053 may wonder how we could have been so interested in serotonin and dopamine in 2003 when many hundreds of more important factors remained to be found.

References

1. Watson JD, Crick FHC: Molecular structure of nucleic acids: a structure for deoxyribose nucleic acid. Nature 1953; 171:737–738
2. Guttmacher AE, Collins FS: Genomic medicine–a primer. N Engl J Med 2002; 347:1512–1519
3. Human Genome Consortium: Initial sequencing and analysis of the human genome. Nature 2001; 409:860–921
4. Venter JC et al: The sequence of the human genome. Science 2001; 291:1304–1351
5. Mouse Genome Sequencing Consortium: Initial sequencing and comparative analysis of the mouse genome. Nature 2002; 420:520–562
6. C. elegans Sequencing Consortium: Genome sequence of pre-nematode C. elegans: a platform for investigating biology. Science 1998; 282:2012–2018
7. Adams MD, Celniker SE, Holt RA, Evans CE, Gocayne JD, et al: The genome sequence of Drosophila melanogaster. Science 2000; 287:2185–2195
8. Graveley BR: Alternative splicing: increased diversity in the proteomic world. Trends Genet 2001; 17:100–107
9. Online Mendelian Inheritance in Man, OMIM ™. Baltimore, McKusick-Nathans Institute for Genetic Medicine, Johns Hopkins University, 2000 (accessed October 15, 2002, at http://www.ncbi.nlm.nih.gov/omim/)
10. Knoers NVAM, Deen PMT: Molecular and cellular defects in nephrogenic diabetes insipidus. Pediatr Nephrol 2001; 16:1146–1152
11. Tanzi RE, Bertram L: New frontiers in Alzheimer's disease genetics. Neuron 2001; 32:181–184
12. Roses AD: Alzheimer diseases: a model of gene mutations and susceptibility polymorphisms for complex psychiatric diseases. Am J Med Genet 1998; 81:49–57

13. Szudek J, Joe H, Friedman JM: Analysis of intrafamilial phenotypic variation in neurofibromatosis 1 (NF1). Genet Epidemiol 2000; 23:150–164

14. Sandberg R, Yasuda R, Pankratz DG, Carter TA, Del Rio JA, Wodicka L, Mayford M, Lockhart DJ, Barlow C: Regional and strain-specific gene expression mapping in the adult mouse brain. Proc Natl Acad Sci USA 2000; 97:11038–11043

15. Maestrini E, Paul A, Monaco AP, Bailey A: Identifying autism susceptibility genes. Neuron 2000, 28:19–24

16. Gottesmann II, Gould TD: The endophenotype concept in psychiatry: etymology and strategic intentions. Am J Psychiatry 2003; 160:636–645

17. Stefansson H, Sigurdsson E, Steinthorsdottir V, Bjornsdottir S, Sigmundsson T, Ghosh S, Brynjolfsson J, Gunnarsdottir S, Ivarsson O, Chou TT, Hjaltason O, Birgisdottir B, Jonsson H, Gudnadottir VG, Gudmundsdottir E, Bjornsson A M, Brunner D, Mutel V, Gonzalo A, Lemke G, Sainz J, Johannesson G, Andresson T, Gudbjartsson D, Manolescu A, Frigge MI, Gurney ME, Kong A, Gulcher JR, Petursson H, Stefansson K: Neuroregulin 1 and susceptibility to schizophrenia. Am J Hum Genet 2002; 71:877–892

18. Stefansson H, Sarginson J, Kong A, Yates P, Steinthorsdottir V, Gudfinnsson E, Gunnarsdottir S, Walker N, Petursson H, Crombie C, Ingason A, Gulcher AR, Stefansson K, Clair DS: Association of neuregulin 1 with schizophrenia confirmed in a Scottish population. Am J Hum Genet 2003; 72:83–87

19. Schwab SG, Knapp M, Mondabon S, Hallmayer J, Borrman-Hassenbach M, Albus M, Lerer B, Rietschel M, Trixler M, Maier W, Wildenauer DB: Support for association of schizophrenia with genetic variation in the 6p22.3 gene, dysbindin, in sib-pair families with linkage and in an additional sample of triad families. Am J Hum Genet 2003; 72:185–190

20. Straub Re, Jiang Y, MacLean CJ, Ma Y, Webb BT, Myakishev MV, Harris-Kerr C, Wormley B, Sadek H, Kadambi B, Cesare AJ, Gibberman A, Wang X: Genetic variation in the 6p22.3 gene DTNBP1, the human ortholog of the mouse dysbindin gene, is associated with schizophrenia. Am J Hum Genet 2002; 71:337–348

21. Chumakov I, Blumenfeld M, Guerassimenko O, Cavarec L, Palicio M, Abderrahim H, Bougueleret L, Barry C, Tanaka H, La Rosa P, Puech A, Tahri N, Cohen-Akenine A, Delabrosse S, Lissarrague S, Picard FP, Maurice K, Essioux L, Millasseau P, Grel P, Debailleul V, Simon AM, Caterina D, Dufaure I, Malekzadeh K, Belova M, Luan JJ, Bouillot M, Sambucy JL, Primas Gsaumier M, Boubkiri N, Martin-Saumier S, Nasroune M, Peixoto H, Delaye A, Pinchot V, Bastucci M, Guillou S, Chevillon M, Sainz-Fuertes R, Meguenni S, Aurich-Costa J, Cherif D, Gimalac A, Van Duijn C, Gauvreau D, Ouellette G, Fortier I, Raelson J, Sherbatich T, Riazanskaia N, Rogaev E, Raeymaekers P, Aerssens J, Konings F, Luyten W, Macciardi F, Sham PC, Straub RE, Weinberger DR, Cohen N, Cohen D, Ouelette G, Raelson J: Genetic and physiological data implicating the new human gene G72 and the gene for D-amino acid oxidase in schizophrenia. Proc Natl Acad Sci USA 2002; 99:13675–13680

22. Egan MF, Goldberg TE, Kolachana BS, Callicott JH, Mazzanti CM, Straub RE, Goldman D, Weinberger DR: Effect of COMT Val108/158 Met genotype on frontal lobe function and risk for schizophrenia. Proc Natl Aca Sci USA 2001; 98:6917–6922

23. Cowan WM, Kopnisky KL, Hyman SE: The human genome project and its impact on psychiatry. Ann Rev Neurosci 2002, 25:1–50

24. Lifton RP, Gharavi AG, Geller DS: Molecular mechanisms of human hypertension. Cell 2001; 104:545–556

25. Gretarsdottir S, Sveinbjornsdottir S, Jonsson HH, Jakobsson F, Einarsdottir E, Agnarsson U, Shkolny D, Einarsson G, Gudjonsdottir HM, Valimarsson EM, Einarsson OB, Thorgeirsson G, Hadzic R, Jonsdottir S, Reynisdottir ST, Bjarnadottir SM, Gudmundsdottir T, Gudlaugsdottir GJ, Gill R, Lindpaintner K, Sainz J, Hannesson HH, Sigurdsson GT, Frigge ML, Kong A, Gudnason V, Stefansson K, Gulcher JR: Localization of a susceptibility gene for common forms of stroke to 5q12. Am J Hum Genet 2002; 70:593–603

26. Caspi A, McClay J, Moffitt TE, Mill J, Martin J, Craig IW, Taylor A, Poulton R: Role of genotype in the cycle of violence in maltreated children. Science 2002; 297:851–853

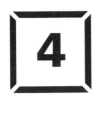

4 | Will the Genomics Revolution Revolutionize Psychiatry?

Kathleen Ries Merikangas, Ph.D.
Neil Risch, Ph.D.

At the time DNA was discovered 50 years ago, psychiatric genetics was in a state of relative dormancy, resulting from the misuse of genetic theories during the World War II era. As the excitement generated by the "new genetics" spread across medical specialty areas, the second half of the century was declared the century of the biological sciences, and genetics research blossomed.[1] Dismissing the widespread notion of a basic conflict between human genetics and religious tenets, Pope Pius XII gave a policy-setting address in 1953, encouraging the need for systematic and ideologically unshackled research in human genetics.[1] In the same year as the discovery of DNA, Franz Kallman's review of progress in psychiatric genetics, published in *The American Journal of Psychiatry*, described a sophisticated series of twin and family studies in the United States[1–3] and Europe[4,5] that corroborated the genetic roots of schizophrenia and manic depressive psychosis that had been demonstrated in the early part of the 20th century. Subsequent research has continued to expand our knowledge of the genetics of psychiatric disorders. As the classification system has grown more specific, genetic investigations have continued to demonstrate the importance of familial and genetic factors underlying most of the major psychiatric conditions.

Overview of Progress in Genetics of Psychiatric Disorders

The wealth of data from family, twin, and adoption studies of the major mental disorders exceeds that of all other chronic human diseases.[1-5] The increased recognition of the role of biologic and genetic vulnerability factors for mental disorders has led to research with increasing methodologic sophistication that has spanned the second half of the 20th century.[6-15] There are numerous comprehensive reviews of genetic research on specific disorders of interest as well as on psychiatric genetics in general.[16-38]

Table 1. Relative risks[a] for selected psychiatric disorders

Disorder	Risk ratio	Heritability estimate
Mood disorders		
Bipolar disorder	7–10	0.60–0.70
Major depression	2–3	0.28–0.40
Anxiety		
All	4–6	0.30–0.40
Panic disorder	3–8	0.50–0.60
Autism	50–100	0.90
Schizophrenia	8–10	0.80–0.84
Substance dependence	4–8	0.30–0.50

[a]Proportion of affected first-degree relatives of affected probands versus the proportion of affected relatives of nonaffected control subjects.

Table 1 presents the relative risks (i.e., proportion affected among first-degree relatives of affected probands versus those of relatives of nonaffected control subjects) derived from controlled family studies of selected psychiatric disorders. The risk ratios comparing the proportion of affected relatives of cases versus control subjects are greatest for autism, bipolar disorder, and schizophrenia; intermediate for substance dependence and subtypes of anxiety, particularly panic; and lowest for major depression. While family studies indicate the degree to which diseases aggregate in families, they alone cannot address the question of genetic versus environmental factors as the source of such aggregation. For this assessment, unusual relationships such as twins, adoptees, or half siblings are required. Estimates of heritability (i.e., the proportion of variance attributable to genetic factors) derived from twin studies, which compare rates of disorders in monozygotic and dizygotic twins, reinforce the notion that genes play a major role in the extent to which mental disorders run in families. The heritability estimates for specific disorders shown in Table 1 are parallel to the risk ratios derived from family studies. Furthermore, adoption and half-sibling studies also support a genetic basis for the observed familial aggregation.[17]

An illustration of the application of family, twin, and adoption study research in psychiatry is provided by bipolar disorder, which is one of the most widely studied psychiatric disorders from a genetic perspective.[22, 39] Recent reviews reveal that the weighted average rate of bipolar disorder among first-degree relatives of bipolar probands is 5.5%, whereas only 0.6% of the relatives of unaffected control subjects have a history of bipolar illness, yielding a risk ratio of 9.2. More refined estimates are available by age, sex, and comorbid disorders in the proband. These estimates can be used to estimate the risk to relatives of individuals with these conditions.

Adoption studies are the most powerful design to test the relative contributions of genetic and environmental factors to etiology. The aggregate adoption study data on mood disorders reveal a moderate increase in rates of mood disorders among biologic compared with adoptive relatives of adoptees with mood disorders.[40] With respect to bipolar disorder, there is little evidence for differential risk among biologic compared with adoptive relatives of adoptees with bipolar disorder. However, the small numbers of bipolar adoptees who have been studied (i.e., less than 50) do not provide an adequate test of genetic and environmental influences.[41] The most compelling finding from adoption studies, however, is the dramatic increase in completed suicide among biological relatives of mood disorder probands.[42, 43]

Methods for Identifying Genes

Linkage and Linkage Disequilibrium

The traditional approach for locating a disease gene in humans is linkage analysis, which tests the association between DNA polymorphic markers and affected status within families. After linkage is detected with an initial marker, many other markers nearby may also be examined. Markers showing the strongest correlation with disease in families are assumed to be closest to the disease locus.

Linkage analysis uses DNA sequences with high variability (i.e., polymorphisms) in order to increase the power to identify markers that are associated with a disease within families. Historically, different methodological approaches have been applied. Earlier linkage studies employed restriction fragment length polymorphisms (RFLPs),[45] whereas subsequent studies examined short tandem repeat markers, or "microsatellites"[46]—DNA sequences that show considerable variability among people but that have no functional consequences. More recently, linkage and association studies have examined single nucleotide polymorphisms (SNPs) to track diseases in families.

Markers in the candidate region identified by linkage analysis can be used to narrow the location of the disease gene through linkage disequilibrium analysis. Linkage disequilibrium is a population association between two alleles at different loci; it occurs when the same founder mutation exists in a large proportion of affected subjects in the population studied. Usually, the closer the marker is to the disease locus, the greater the proportion of affected subjects who carry the identical allele at the marker.[44] However, in measuring the strength of linkage disequilibrium for a given marker, it is also important to select unaffected control subjects from the same population, since an allele shared among affected subjects may also be common in the general population and thus shared by chance rather than due to proximity to the disease locus.[44]

For complex human diseases, a simple mode of genetic inheritance is not apparent, and indeed, multiple contributing genetic loci are likely to be involved. Study designs that do not depend on the particular mode of inheritance are required for linkage analysis. Since affected relatives provide most of the information for such analyses, studies that focus on searching for increased sharing of marker alleles above chance expectation among affected relatives may be employed. The simplest of such studies involves affected sibships, where allele sharing in excess of 50% (the expectation when there is no linkage) is sought.

Association Studies

Linkage analysis has not proven successful in identifying genes for most complex diseases, presumably because the effects of the underlying genes are not strong enough to be detected by linkage.[47] Therefore, genome-wide association studies have been offered as a more powerful approach. Completion of the human genome project has provided an unprecedented opportunity to identify the effect of gene variants on complex phenotypes, such as psychiatric disorders. Functional genomics technology involving microarrays and proteomics will provide added insights regarding gene function on the cellular level, improving our ability to predict phenotypic effects of genes at the organismic level.[44] The recently proposed project (known as the HapMap project) to develop a map of human haplotypes, or blocks of genes that may have been conserved in evolutionary history, has generated considerable enthusiasm for its potential to inform the genetic basis of complex disorders in the general population. There has been considerable discussion regarding the value of studying SNPs with functional significance[47] versus noncoding or evenly spaced SNPs.[48] Botstein and Risch[49] have proposed that the initial work employ sequence-based association studies that focus on functional coding regions, rather than a map-based approach[48, 50, 51] that relies solely on the location of haplotypes in order to maximize power and efficiency for the detection of genes for complex human diseases.

Association studies examine candidate genes among affected individuals and unrelated unaffected control subjects. The same limitations that apply to case-control studies of other risk factors must also be considered in genetic case-control studies. The most serious problem in the design of association studies is the failure to select control subjects who are comparable to the cases on all factors except the disease of interest. Failure to equate cases and control subjects may lead to confounding (i.e., a spurious association due to an unmeasured factor that is associated with both the candidate gene and the disease). In genetic case-control studies, the most likely source of confounding is ethnicity because of differential gene and disease frequencies in different ethnic subgroups. Aside from confounding, association studies are particularly prone to false positive findings due to multiple testing without correction and the low prior probability of a gene-disease association.[52, 53] The latter problem can be resolved in part by the use of more stringent alpha levels (i.e., false positive error rates) in association studies.[47] In addition, there is a strong publication bias against reports of negative association studies.[54]

The Importance of Replication

Within the past two decades, linkage analysis has had remarkable success in identifying genes for Mendelian diseases such as cystic fibrosis and Huntington's disease, among many others. Several of these genes also account for an uncommon subset of generally more common disorders such as breast cancer (BRCA1 and 2), colon cancer (familial adenomatous polyposis), hereditary nonpolyposis colorectal cancer, and Alzheimer's disease (β-amyloid precursor protein and presenilin-1 and -2).

Despite these successes, linkage studies of complex disorders have been difficult to replicate. A recent review of the linkage findings for 31 complex human diseases based on whole genome screens concluded that the genetic localization of most susceptibility loci is still imprecise and difficult to replicate.[55] Increased success in the replication of linkage studies was associated with two study features: an increase in the sample size and ethnic homogeneity of the sample.[55] Hirschhorn et al.[54] conducted a similar review of genetic association studies and concluded that few were reproducible. Although these latter reviews do not inspire confidence in the future of these strategies for identifying genes for complex diseases, the studies reviewed still represent the early phases of the application of an extremely powerful technology. Substantial effort will be required to refine phenotypes, identify sources of complexity, and develop new tools and methods to maximize the likelihood of identifying genetic risk factors.

The basis of all scientific research is hypothesis testing and validation of results by independent researchers. Independent replication, typically viewed as the sine qua non for accepting a hypothesis, has become an especially difficult issue in the genetic studies of complex diseases. When a genetic effect is large, most independent researchers can readily obtain similar results with strong levels of statistical significance.[44] Most genes for Mendelian disorders have lived up to this expectation. However, when genetic effects are weak and possibly context-dependent (e.g., they may vary by sex, ethnicity, or precision of diagnosis), replication may be particularly difficult, and very large samples may be required before confident conclusions can be drawn.

Application of Linkage and Association to Psychiatric Disorders

With the aforementioned dramatic advances in molecular genetics during the past 20 years, there has been a major shift in the focus of psychiatric genetic investigations from elucidating patterns of familial transmission to localizing genes underlying mental disorders using linkage studies and, more recently, association studies.[56, 57] The early successes of linkage studies of Mendelian diseases generated a strong sense of optimism that the same approach would be successful for mental disorders and other complex disorders.[58, 59] However, the promise has been unfulfilled to date.[21, 24, 56, 57, 60–65] For example, in a recent summary of genome-wide linkage studies of bipolar disorder based on gene scans in a total of 3,538 affected subjects from 1,119 pedigrees reported in 20 samples, Prathikanti and McMahon[66] concluded that no two studies conclusively implicated the same region. The most striking conclusions were that no two studies employed identical ascertainment procedures and that there was substantial diversity in sampling and methods.

Because of increasing skepticism in accepting the findings of linkage and association studies, there has been considerable debate regarding what constitutes acceptable evidence of a true replication. For example, failure to replicate an initial report of linkage between schizophrenia and a marker on chromosome 1q in 22 families[67, 68] was attributed to study design[67] and heterogeneity,[69] even though the replication study was conducted on a very large sample of 722 families.[70] There have been several recent attempts to standardize the criteria for confirming linkage and association findings.

The ping-pong game between linkage and association claims and disconfirmations has been referred to as a "manic depressive history" by Risch and Botstein.[71] It has been particularly difficult for psychiatric clinicians on the front lines to interpret progress in psychiatric genetics because of the inconsistency of findings as well as the difficulty in comprehending the complex methods of molecular biology and the statistical methods of genetic epidemiology. Nevertheless, there are several recent promising findings in psychiatric genetics described in this book, although replication remains the cornerstone before such findings can be generally accepted. In addition, the increasing tendency for collaborative efforts on genetics studies within psychiatry may also help to offset some of the aforementioned inconsistencies.[35, 70, 72]

Sources of Complexity in Mental Disorders

Two major contributors to the complex patterns of inheritance with regard to psychiatric disorders are 1) the lack of validity of the classification of psychiatric disorders (e.g., phenotypes or observable aspects of diseases) and 2) the complexity of the pathways from genotypes to psychiatric phenotypes.

Lack of Validity of the Classification System

Psychiatric disorder phenotypes, based solely on clinical manifestations without pathognomonic markers, still lack conclusive evidence for the validity of classification and the reliability of measurement.[73]

This situation is not caused by a lack of attention to classification in psychiatry; in fact, advances in the development of standardized classification and assessment methods have superseded those of most other clinically defined diagnostic entities. The development of structured interviews has enhanced comparability of diagnostic methods within the United States and worldwide. There is now an exciting venture designed to collect information on the prevalence of mental disorders which is using comparable diagnostic tools in more than 20 countries under the auspices of the World Mental Health 2000 Initiative (sponsored by the World Health Organization).[74]

The continued reliance on the descriptive approach as the sole basis for diagnosis in psychiatry can be attributed to the greater complexity of the human brain relative to other human systems. In fact, mental disorders involve the highest level of human functioning. Therefore, the difficulty in classifying human cognition, behavior, and emotion is not unexpected in light of the complex psychological and physiological states underlying mental function, which is the product of the entire human experience in adaptation to the environment.[75] Advances in the tools to tap human brain functioning in vivo have led to dramatic advances in knowledge about central nervous system function.[76] However, this work is still in its infancy. These advances are likely to yield valuable information for understanding and, hence, classification of mental disorders.

Complex Patterns of Transmission

The application of advances in genomics to mental disorders is still limited by the complexity of the process through which genes exert their influence. There is substantial evidence that a lack of one-to-one correspondence between the genotype and phenotype exists for most of the major mental disorders. Phenomena such as penetrance (i.e., probability of phenotypic expression among individuals with a susceptibility gene), variable expressivity (i.e., variation in clinical expression associated with a particular gene), gene-environment interaction (i.e., expression of genotype only in the presence of particular environmental exposures), pleiotropy (i.e., capacity of genes to manifest several different phenotypes simultaneously), genetic heterogeneity (i.e., different genes leading to indistinguishable phenotypes), and polygenic and oligogenic modes of inheritance (i.e., simultaneous contributions of multiple genes rather than Mendelian single-gene models) are characteristic of the mental disorders, as they are of numerous other complex disorders for which susceptibility genes have been identified.[77, 78] Other complicated situations include mitochondrial inheritance, imprinting, and other epigenetic phenomena.[79]

The high magnitude of comorbidity and co-aggregation of index disorders with other major psychiatric disorders (i.e., bipolar disorder and alcoholism, major depression and anxiety disorders, schizophrenia and drug dependence), in part induced by the classification system, has been demonstrated in both clinical and community studies.[80-85] For example, alcoholism, a well-established complication of bipolar illness, may mask the underlying features of bipolarity, leading to phenotypic misclassification in genetic studies.[86] Nonrandom mating is also a common phenomenon in mental disorders that impedes evaluation of patterns of familial transmission.[84] Assortative mating is particularly pronounced for substance use disorders for which substance dependence among spouses of substance dependent probands may be as high as 90%.[84, 87] These phenomena serve to increase the noise-to-signal ratio in defining the mental disorders for genetic studies. Studies that attempt to identify the impact of these phenomena on phenotypic and endophenotypic expression in individuals and families will bring us closer to understanding the role of the underlying genes on the components of mental disorders.

Future Research to Resolve Sources of Complexity

Use of Endophenotypes for Classification

With plans for the development of the DSM-V under way, it is essential that scientific evidence be used to revise the diagnostic classification system.[88] There is abundant research on sources of comorbidity, dimensional classification of disorders, and inclusion of subthreshold diagnostic categories and diagnostic spectra.[89-91] As this effort continues, research on the classification of the phenotype for genetic and other biologic studies should increasingly strive for classification that may more closely represent expression of underlying biologic systems.

Phenotypic traits or markers that may represent more direct expressions of underlying genes and the broader disease phenotype have been termed "endophenotypes"[77] (see the review article by Gottesman and Gould in this book). Studies of the role of genetic factors involved in these systems may be far more informative than studies of the aggregate psychiatric phenotypes. Since endophenotypes should more clearly represent expression of genotypes, it is likely that they will help to unravel the complexity of transmission of the mental disorders. Progress in understanding the pathogenesis of the mental disorders and their component features will enhance identification of endophenotypes and provide a more fertile ground for interaction with basic science. For example, some of the endophenotypes that may underlie mood disorders include circadian rhythm, stress reactivity, and mood, sleep, and appetite regulation.[92] Numerous other endophenotypes have also been examined for other disorders, including schizophrenia,[77, 93–95] anxiety disorders,[65] and attention deficit disorder.[96] Some examples of the direct implications of the advances in neuroscience and neuroimaging for phenotypic characterization are described by Thompson et al.[97] and Dolan.[75]

Genetic Epidemiology

Applying the tools of genetic epidemiology, particularly when coupled with continued progress in the neurosciences and behavioral sciences, is likely to be one of the most fruitful approaches to resolving sources of complexity in the mental disorders and translating the progress in genomics to the public.[98] Figure 1 shows the classic triangle that illustrates the major focus of epidemiologic investigations: the products of the interaction between the host, an infectious or other type of agent, and the environment that promotes the exposure.[99] The factors that may be associated with increased risk of human disease are shown under each of the three domains of influence. The field of genetic epidemiology focuses on the role of genetic factors that interact with other domains of risk to enhance vulnerability or protection against disease.[100–102] It is quite conceivable that several combinations of these risk factors could produce similar phenotypes in susceptible individuals. The test for epidemiology over the next decades will be to determine the extent to which the tools can be refined to capture these situations.

Sampling

The shift from systematic large-scale family studies to linkage studies in psychiatry has led to the collection of families according to very specific sampling strategies (e.g., many affected relatives, affected sibling pairs, affected relatives on one side of the family only, availability of parents for study, etc.) in order to maximize the power of detecting genes according to the assumed model of familial transmission. Despite the increase in power for detecting genes, these sampling approaches have diminished the generalizability of the study findings and contribute little else to the knowledge base if genes are not discovered. As we learn more about the complexity of genetic risk factors, it may be advisable in the fu-

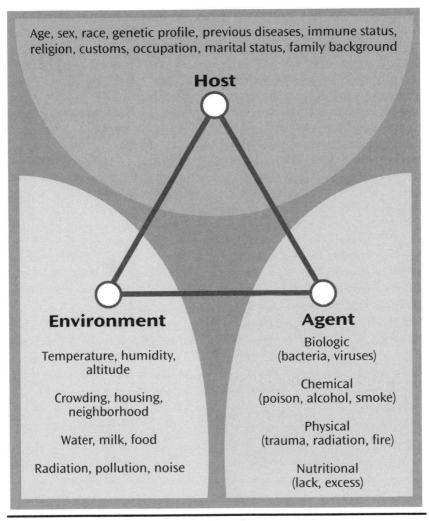

Figure 1. The Epidemiologic Triangle

ture to collect both families and control subjects from representative samples of the population in order to enable estimation of population risk parameters, enhance generalizability, and examine the specificity of endophenotypic transmission.

Study Designs

Epidemiologic studies generally proceed from retrospective case-control studies to develop specific hypotheses that can be addressed in prospective cohort studies in order to demonstrate causality. The major goal of analytic epidemiology is to identify risk and protective factors and their causal links to disease, with the ultimate goal of disease prevention. Genetic epidemiology employs traditional epidemiologic study designs to identify explanatory factors for aggregation in groups of relatives ranging from twins to migrant cohorts. The tools of genetic epidemiology will be employed in the era of genomics to derive estimates of the population distribution of disease genes, to test modes of disease transmission in systematic samples that are representative of the population, and to identify sources of gene-environment interactions for diseases. Since epidemiology has developed sophisticated designs and analytic methods for identifying disease risk factors, these methods can now be extended to include both genes and environmental factors as gene identification proceeds.

In general, study designs in genetic epidemiology either control for genetic background while letting the environment vary (e.g., migrant studies, half siblings, separated twins) or control for the environment while allowing variance in the genetic background (e.g., siblings, twins, adoptees-nonbiological siblings). Because each of the study designs has both strengths and limitations, it is important to evaluate aggregate evidence from multiple approaches to yield conclusive evidence regarding the role of genetic and environmental risk factors. Over the next decades, it will be important to identify and evaluate the effects of specific environmental factors on disease outcomes and to refine measurement of environmental exposures to evaluate specificity of effects.

Migrant studies are perhaps the most powerful study design to identify environmental and cultural risk factors. One of the earliest controlled migrant studies evaluated rates of psychosis among Norwegian immigrants to Minnesota compared with native Minnesotans and native Norwegians.[103] The higher rate of psychosis among the immigrants than in both the native Minnesotans and Norwegians was attributed to greater susceptibility to psychosis among the migrants who left Norway. It was found that migration selection bias was the major explanatory factor rather than an environmental exposure in the new culture.[103]

Another powerful study design is the nested case-control study built on an established cohort. Prospective cohort studies are also valuable sources of diagnostic stability, causal associations between risk factors and disease, and developmental aspects of psychiatric disorders. Langholz et al.[104] described some of the world's prospective cohort studies that may serve as a basis for studies of gene-disease associations or gene-environment interactions. Finally, the half-sibling approach may eventually replace the adoption paradigm to investigate genetic and environmental effects because of the recent trends toward selective adoption and the diminishing frequency of adoptions in the United States and in numerous other countries (i.e., maternal selection of adoptive parents and continued contact with biological mothers).

Population-Based Studies

The importance of epidemiology to the future of genetics has been described by numerous geneticists and epidemiologists who conclude that the best strategy for gene identification will ultimately involve large epidemiologic studies from diverse populations.[39, 44, 47, 98, 105–108] It is likely that population-based association studies will assume increasing importance in translating the products of genomics to public health.[47] The term "human genome epidemiology" was coined by Khoury et al.[108] to denote the emerging field that employs systematic applications of epidemiologic methods in population-based studies of the impact of human genetic variation on health and disease.

There are several reasons that population-based studies will be critical to the future of genetics. First, the prevalence of newly identified polymorphisms, whether SNPs or other variants, especially in particular population subgroups, is not known. Second, current knowledge of genes as risk factors is based nearly exclusively on clinical and nonsystematic samples. Hence, the significance of the susceptibility alleles that have been identified for cancer, heart disease, diabetes, and so forth is unknown in the population at large. In order to provide accurate risk estimates, the next stage of research needs to move beyond samples identified through affected individuals to the population in order to obtain estimates of the risk of specific polymorphisms for the population as a whole. Third, identification of risk profiles will require very large samples to assess the significance of vulnerability genes with relatively low expected population frequencies. Fourth, similar to the role of epidemiology in quantifying risk associated with traditional disease risk factors, applications of human genome epidemiology can provide information on the specificity, sensitivity, and impact of genetic tests to inform science and the individual.[107]

Because genetic polymorphisms involved in complex diseases are likely to be nondeterministic (i.e., the marker neither predicts disease nor nondisease with certainty), traditional epidemiologic risk factor designs can be used to estimate their impact.[101] As epidemiologists add genes to their risk equations, it is likely that the contradictory findings from studies that have generally employed solely environmental risk factors, such as diet, smoking, alcohol use, etc., will be resolved. Likewise, the studies that seek solely to identify genes will also continue to be inconsistent without considering the effects of nongenetic biologic parameters as well as environmental factors that contribute to the diseases of interest.

There are several types of risk estimates that are used in public health. The most common is relative risk, the magnitude of the association between an exposure and disease. It is independent of the prevalence of the exposure. The absolute risk is the overall probability of developing a disease in a particular population.[99] The population attributable risk relates to the risk of a disease in a total population (exposed and unexposed) and indicates the amount the disease can be reduced in a population if an exposure were eliminated. The population attributable risk depends on the prevalence of the exposure, or in the case of genes, the gene frequency. Genetic attributable risk would indicate the proportion of a particular disease that may be attributed to a particular genetic locus.

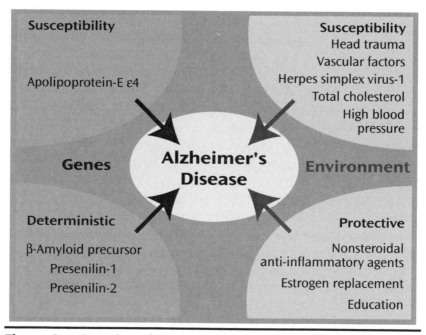

Figure 2.   Genetic and environmental factors in Alzheimer's disease

Figure 2 illustrates the known genetic and environmental risk factors for Alzheimer's disease.[109] The orange areas on the left represent the roles of deterministic genes (β-amyloid precursor, presenilin-1 and -2) and the susceptibility gene apolipoprotein-E ε4 (APOE ε4).[110] The blue areas on the right indicate environmental risk and protective factors, respectively.[111-113] Individuals with mutations in deterministic genes appear to have nearly a 100% chance (i.e., fully penetrant) for the development of Alzheimer's disease. Likewise, the relative risk of these genes would also be quite high. In contrast, because these mutations are presumed to be very rare in the population, the population attributable risk is quite low, meaning that were these mutations to be eliminated from the population, there would be little impact on the prevalence of Alzheimer's disease.

The APOE ε4 allele has been shown to increase the risk of Alzheimer's disease in a dose-dependent fashion. Using data from a large multiethnic sample collected by more than 40 research teams, Farrer et al.[114] reported a 2.6–3.2 greater odds of Alzheimer's disease among those with one copy, and 14.9 odds of Alzheimer's disease among those with two copies of the APOE ε4 allele. Moreover, there was a significant protective effect among those with the ε2/ε3 genotype. As opposed to the deterministic mutations, the APOE ε4 allele has a very high population attributable risk because of its high frequency in the population.

Identification of Environmental Factors

The identification of gene-environment interactions will be one of the most important future goals of genetic epidemiology. Newman et al.[115] credit the synergy between genetics and epidemiology for elucidating the initial gene findings as well as for the subsequent identification of other susceptibility alleles and the environmental factors that may influence the risk of breast cancer in susceptible persons. Study designs and statistical methods should focus increasingly on gene-environment interaction.[116-122] Evidence is emerging that gene-environment interaction underlies many of the complex human diseases. Some examples include inborn errors of metabolism, individual variation in response to drugs,[123] substance use disorders,[124, 125] and the protective influence of a deletion in the CCR5 gene on exposure to HIV.[79, 126]

With respect to mental disorders, recent reviews of prospective studies that evaluated environmental risk factors for the common mental disorders ascertained in population-based studies yielded few specific environmental factors that could be etiologically linked with any of the major mental disorders.[127] However, one promising exception is the increasing evidence from genetic epidemiologic studies that environmental exposures including pre- and perinatal factors, such as viral agents, may enhance the risk of schizophrenia.[128] Other informative study designs for identifying gene-environment interactions include migrant studies and genetic case-control studies in which the cases may be defined by a genetic susceptibility marker.

Future research designed to identify environmental factors that operate either specifically or nonspecifically on those with susceptibility to mental disorders may provide an important opportunity for prevention and intervention, once susceptibility genes have been identified. The recent advances in understanding the bidirectional communication of neural systems and experience[76] provide an ideal opportunity to apply genetic epidemiologic methods such as case-control and prospective cohort studies. Increased knowledge of the developmental pathways of emotion, cognition, and behavior will expand our ability to identify specific environmental factors such as infection, poor diet, prenatal environment, and early life experiences that interact with the genetic architecture of mood regulation and cognition.[129]

Impact of Genomics on Psychiatric Science and Practice

Will genomics lead to changes in medical practice and transform psychiatric genetics?

In a recent summary of implications of the genome for medical practice, Varmus[130] concluded that despite the journalistic hyperbole, the sequencing of the human genome is unlikely to lead to either a radical transformation of medical practice or even to an information-based science that can predict with certainty future diseases and effective treatment interventions. Although this skepticism may be somewhat extreme, it is clear that progress in genomics has far outweighed advances in our understanding of psychiatric phenotypes and the complexity underlying their etiology, as well as our current armamentarium to identify genetic and environmental risk factors. Therefore, despite the extraordinary opportunity for understanding disease pathogenesis afforded by the technical advances and availability of rapidly expanding genetic databases, it is unlikely that we will soon experience the light speed progress of genomics in understanding, treating, or preventing major mental disorders. The chasm between genetic information and clinical utility should gradually close as we develop new methods and tools in human genetic and clinical research to maximize the knowledge afforded by the exciting advances in genomics.

Increased integration of advances in neuroscience[131] and genomics (see the series of papers in the *New England Journal of Medicine* such as the primer by Guttmacher and Collins[79]), along with information from population-based studies and longitudinal cohorts, innovations in our conceptualizations of the mental disorders, and the identification of specific risk and protective factors, will lead to more informed intervention strategies in psychiatry. As we learn more about the role of genes as risk factors, rather than as the chief causes of common human diseases, it will be essential to provide accurate risk estimation and to inform the public of the need for population-based integrated data on genetic, biologic, and environmental risk factors.

The goal of genomics research is ultimately prevention, the cornerstone of public health. Gaining understanding of the significance of genetic risk factors and learning proper interpretation of their meaning for patients and their families will ultimately become part of clinical practice, and clinicians will be involved more than ever in helping patients to comprehend the meaning and potential impact of genetic risk for nonpsychiatric disorders as well. As our knowledge on the role of genes for mental disorders advances, it will be incumbent upon clinicians to become familiar with knowledge gleaned from genetic epidemiologic and genomics research. In the meanwhile, recurrence risk estimates from family studies constitute the best available knowledge on which to predict the risk of the development of mental disorders.

References

1. Kallmann FJ: Review of psychiatric progress 1953. Am J Psychiatry 1954; 110:489–492
2. Kallmann FJ, Jarvik LF: Individual differences in constitution and genetic background, in Aging and the Individual. Edited by Birren JE. Chicago, University of Chicago Press, 1959
3. Stenstedt A: A study in manic-depressive psychosis: clinical, social, and genetic investigations. Acta Psychiatr Neurol Scand 1952; 42:398–409
4. Slater E: The incidence of mental disorder. Annals of Eugenics 1935; 6:172
5. Böök JA: A genetic and neuropsychiatric investigation of a north-Swedish population with special regard to schizophrenia and mental deficiency. Acta Genet Stat Med 1953; 4:70–84
6. Reich T, Clayton PJ, Winokur G: Family history studies, V: the genetics of mania. Am J Psychiatry 1969; 125:1358–1369
7. Tsuang M, Dempsey G, Dvoredsky A, Strauss A: A family history study of schizoaffective disorder. Biol Psychiatry 1977; 12:331–338
8. Winokur G, Tsuang MT, Crowe RR: The Iowa 500: affective disorder in relatives of manic and depressed patients. Am J Psychiatry 1982; 139:209–212
9. Andreasen NC, Rice J, Endicott J, Coryell W, Grove WM, Reich T: Familial rates of affective disorder: a report from the National Institute of Mental Health Collaborative Study. Arch Gen Psychiatry 1987; 44:461–469; correction, 1988; 45:776

10. Gershon ES, Hamovit J, Guroff JJ: A family study of schizoaffective, bipolar I, bipolar II, unipolar, and normal control probands. Arch Gen Psychiatry 1982; 39:1157–1167

11. Weissman MM, Kidd KK, Prusoff BA: Variability in rates of affective disorders in relatives of depressed and normal probands. Arch Gen Psychiatry 1982; 39:1397–1403

12. Kendler KS: Twin studies of psychiatric illness: an update. Arch Gen Psychiatry 2001; 58:1005–1014

13. Kety SS, Rosenthal D, Wender PH, Schulsinger F: The types of prevalence of mental illness in the biological and adoptive families of adopted schizophrenics, in The Transmission of Schizophrenia. Edited by Rosenthal D, Kety SS. Oxford, UK, Pergamon Press, 1968

14. Rosenthal D: Some factors associated with concordance and discordance with respect to schizophrenia in monozygotic twins. J Nerv Ment Dis 1959; 129:1–10

15. Weissman MM, Gershon ES, Kidd KK, Prusoff BA, Leckman JF, Dibble E, Hamovit JH, Thompson WD, Pauls DL, Guroff JJ: Psychiatric disorder in relatives of probands with affective disorders: the Yale University-NIMH Collaborative Family Study. Arch Gen Psychiatry 1984; 41:13–21

16. Plomin R, Defries JC, McClearn GE, McGuffin F: Behavioral Genetics. London, WH Freeman and Company, 2000

17. Merikangas KR, Swendsen JD: Genetic epidemiology of psychiatric disorders. Epidemiol Rev 1996; 19:1–12

18. McGuffin P, Owen MJ, Gottesman II: Psychiatric Genetics and Genomics. Oxford, UK, Oxford University Press, 2002

19. Moldin SO: Summary of research—appendix to the report of the NIMH's Genetics Workgroup. Biol Psychiatry 1999; 45:573–602

20. McGuffin P, Asherson P, Owen M, Farmer A: The strength of the genetic effect: is there room for an environmental influence in the aetiology of schizophrenia? Br J Psychiatry 1994; 164:593–599

21. Craddock N, Jones I: Molecular genetics of bipolar disorder. Br J Psychiatry Suppl 2001; 41:S128–S133

22. Sullivan PF, Neale MC, Kendler KS: Genetic epidemiology of major depression: review and meta-analysis. Am J Psychiatry 2000; 157:1552–1562

23. Kendler KS, Neale MC, Kessler RC: Panic disorder in women: a population-based twin study. Psychol Med 1993; 23:397–406

24. van den Heuvel OA, van de Wetering BJ, Veltman DJ, Pauls DL: Genetic studies of panic disorder: a review. J Clin Psychiatry 2000; 61:756–766

25. Smoller JW, Finn C, White C: The genetics of anxiety disorders: an overview. Psychiatr Annals 2000; 30:745–753

26. Nestadt G, Samuels J, Riddle M, Bienvenu OJI, Liang K-Y, LaBuda M, Walkup J, Grados M, Hoehn-Saric R: A family study of obsessive-compulsive disorder. Arch Gen Psychiatry 2000; 57:358–363

27. Sullivan PF, Kendler KS: Typology of common psychiatric syndromes: an empirical study. Br J Psychiatry 1998; 173:312–319

28. Kendler KS, Prescott CA: Cannabis use, abuse, and dependence in a population-based sample of female twins. Am J Psychiatry 1998; 155:1016–1022

29. Kendler K, Prescott C: Cocaine use, abuse and dependence in a population-based sample of female twins. Br J Psychiatry 1998; 173:345–350

30. Merikangas KR: Genetic epidemiology of substance-use disorders, in Textbook of Biological Psychiatry. Edited by D'haenen, Den Boer J, Willner P. New York, John Wiley & Sons, 2002, pp 537–546

31. Uhl GR, Liu QR, Naiman D: Substance abuse vulnerability loci: converging genome scanning data. Trends Genet 2002; 18:420–425

32. Rice F, Harold G, Thapar A: The genetic aetiology of childhood depression: a review. J Child Psychol Psychiatry 2002; 43:65–79

33. Szatmari P, Jones MB, Zwaigenbaum L, MacLean JE: Genetics of autism: overview and new directions. J Autism Dev Disord 1998; 28:351–368

34. Risch N, Spiker D, Lotspeich L, Nouri N, Hinds D, Hallmayer J, Kalaydjieva L, McCague P, Dimiceli S, Pitts T, Nguyen L, Yang J, Harper C, Thorpe D, Vermeer S, Young H, Hebert J, Lin A, Ferguson J, Chiotti C, Wiese-Slater S, Rogers T, Salmon B, Nicholas P, Myers RM, et al: A genomic screen of autism: evidence for a multilocus etiology. Am J Hum Genet 1999; 65:493–507

35. International Molecular Genetic Study of Autism Consortium: A full genome screen for autism with evidence for linkage to a region on chromosome 7q. Hum Mol Genet 1998; 7:571–578

36. Thapar A, Holmes J, Poulton K, Harrington R: Genetic basis of attention deficit and hyperactivity. Br J Psychiatry 1999; 174:105–111

37. Thapar A, Scourfield J: Childhood disorders, in Psychiatric Genetics and Genomics. Edited by McGuffin P, Owen MJ, Gottesman II. Oxford, UK, Oxford University Press, 2002, pp 147–180

38. Rutter M, Silberg J, O'Connor T, Simonoff E: Genetics and child psychiatry, II: empirical research findings. J Child Psychol Psychiatry 1999; 40:19–55

39. Merikangas KR, Chakravarti A, Moldin SO, Araj H, Blangero J, Burmeister M, Crabbe JCJ, DePaulo JRJ, Foulks E, Freimer NB, Koretz DS, Lichtenstein W, Mignot E, Reiss AL, Risch NJ, Takahashi J (Workgroup on Genetics for NIMH Strategic Plan for Mood Disorders): Future of genetics of mood disorders research. Biol Psychiatry 2002; 52:457–477

40. Tsuang MT, Faraone SV: The Genetics of Mood Disorders. Baltimore, Johns Hopkins University Press, 1990

41. Goodwin FK, Jamison KR: Manic-Depressive Illness. New York, Oxford University Press, 1990

42. Wender PH, Kety SS, Rosenthal D, Schulsinger F, Ortmann J, Lunde I: Psychiatric disorders in the biological and adoptive families of adopted individuals with affective disorders. Arch Gen Psychiatry 1986; 43:923–929

43. Mendlewicz J, Rainer JD: Adoption study supporting genetic transmission in manic-depressive illness. Nature 1977; 268:326–329
44. Risch NJ: Searching for genetic determinants in the new millennium. Nature 2000; 405:847–856
45. Botstein D, White RL, Skolnick M, Davis RW: Construction of a genetic linkage map in man using restriction fragment length polymorphisms. Am J Hum Genet 1980; 32:314–331
46. Weber JL, May PE: Abundant class of human DNA polymorphisms which can be typed using the polymerase chain reaction. Am J Hum Genet 1989; 44:388–396
47. Risch N, Merikangas KR: The future of genetic studies of complex human diseases. Science 1996; 273:1516–1517
48. Collins FS, Guyer MS, Charkravarti A: Variations on a theme: cataloging human DNA sequence variation. Science 1997; 278:1580–1581
49. Botstein D, Risch N: Discovering genotypes underlying human phenotypes: past successes for mendelian disease, future approaches for complex disease. Nat Genet Suppl 2003; 33
50. Patil N: Blocks of limited haplotype diversity revealed by high-resolution scanning of human chromosome 21. Science 2001; 294:1719–1723
51. Gabriel SB: The structure of haplotype blocks in the human genome. Science 2002; 296:2225–2228
52. Wacholder S, Rothman N, Caporaso N: Population stratification in epidemiologic studies of common genetic variants and cancer: quantification of bias. J Natl Cancer Inst 2000; 92:1151–1158
53. Wacholder S, Garcia-Closas M, Rothman N: Study of genes and environmental factors in complex diseases (letter). Lancet 2002; 359:1155
54. Hirschhorn JN, Lohmueller K, Byrne E, Hirschhorn K: A comprehensive review of genetic association studies. Genet Med 2002; 4:45–61
55. Altmuller J, Palmer LJ, Fischer G, Scherb H, Wjst M: Genomewide scans of complex human diseases: true linkage is hard to find. Am J Hum Genet 2001; 69:936–950
56. McInnes LA, Freimer NB: Mapping genes for psychiatric disorders and behavioral traits. Curr Opin Genet Dev 1995; 5:376–381
57. DeLisi LE, Craddock NJ, Detera-Wadleigh S, Foroud T, Gejman P, Kennedy JL, Lendon C, Macciardi F, McKeon P, Mynett-Johnson L, Nurnberger JI Jr, Paterson A, Schwab S, Van Broeckhoven C, Wildenauer D, Crow TJ: Update on chromosomal locations for psychiatric disorders: report of the interim meeting of chromosome workshop chairpersons from the VIIth World Congress of Psychiatric Genetics, Monterey, California, October 14–18, 1999. Am J Med Genet 2000; 96:434–449
58. Risch N: Searching for genes in complex diseases: lessons from systemic lupus erythematosus. J Clin Invest 2000; 105:1503–1506
59. Glazier AM, Nadeau JH, Aitman TJ: Finding genes that underlie complex traits. Science 2002; 298:2345–2349

60. Moises HW, Yang L, Kristbjarnarson H, Wiese C, Byerley W, Macciardi F, Arolt V, Blackwood D, Liu X, Sjogren B, et al: An international two-stage genome-wide search for schizophrenia susceptibility genes. Nat Genet 1995; 11:321–324

61. Faraone SV, Matise T, Svrakic D, Pepple J, Malaspina D, Suarez B, Hampe C, Zambuto CT, Schmitt K, Meyer J, Markel P, Lee H, Harkavy Friedman J, Kaufmann C, Cloninger CR, Tsuang MT: Genome scan of European-American schizophrenia pedigrees: results of the NIMH Genetics Initiative and Millennium Consortium. Am J Med Genet 1998; 81:290–295

62. O'Donovan MC, Owen MJ: Candidate-gene association studies of schizophrenia. Am J Hum Genet 1999; 65:587–592

63. Riley BP, McGuffin P: Linkage and associated studies of schizophrenia. Am J Med Genet 2000; 97:23–44

64. Sklar P: Linkage analysis in psychiatric disorders: the emerging picture. Annu Rev Genomics Hum Genet 2002; 3:371–413

65. Smoller JW, Tsuang MT: Panic and phobic anxiety: defining phenotypes for genetic science. Am J Psychiatry 1998; 155:1152–1162

66. Prathikanti S, McMahon FJ: Genome scans for susceptibility genes in bipolar affective disorder. Ann Med 2001; 33:257–262

67. Bassett AS, Chow EW, Vieland VJ, Brzustowicz L: Is schizophrenia linked to chromosome 1q? (letter). Science 2002; 298:2277

68. Brzustowicz LM, Hodgkinson KA, Chow EW, Honer WG, Bassett AS: Location of a major susceptibility locus for familial schizophrenia on chromosome 1q21-q22. Science 2000; 288:678–682

69. Macgregor S, Visscher PM, Knott S, Porteous D, Muir W, Millar K, Blackwood D: Is schizophrenia linked to chromosome 1q? (letter). Science 2002; 298:2277

70. Levinson DF, Holmans PA, Laurent C, Riley B, Pulver AE, Gejman PV, Schwab SG, Williams NM, Owen MJ, Wildenauer DB, Sanders AR, Nestadt G, Mowry BJ, Wormley B, Bauche S, Soubigou S, Ribble R, Nertney DA, Liang KY, Martinolich L, Maier W, Norton N, Williams H, Albus M, Carpenter EB, DeMarchi N, Ewen-White KR, Walsh D, Jay M, Deleuze JF, O'Neill FA, Papadimitriou G, Weilbaecher A, Lerer B, O'Donovan MC, Dikeos D, Silverman JM, Kendler KS, Mallet J, Crowe RR, Walters M: No major schizophrenia locus detected on chromosome 1q in a large multicenter sample. Science 2002; 296:739–741

71. Risch N, Botstein DA: A manic depressive history. Nat Genet 1996; 12:351–353

72. Detera-Wadleigh SD, Badner JA, Berrettini WH, Yoshikawa T, Goldin LR, Turner G: A high-density genome scan detects evidence for a bipolar-disorder susceptibility locus on 13q32 and other potential loci on 1q32 and 18p11.2. Proc Natl Acad Sci USA 1999; 96:5604–5609

73. Kendell RE: Clinical validity. Psychol Med 1989; 19:45–55

74. Kessler RC, Üstün TB: The World Health Organization World Mental Health 2000 Initiative. Hosp Management Int 2000:195–196

75. Dolan RJ: Emotion, cognition, and behavior. Science 2002; 298:1191–1194
76. McKhann GM: Neurology: then, now, and in the future. Arch Neurol 2002; 59:1369–1373
77. Gottesman I, Shields J: Schizophrenia and Genetics: A Twin Study Vantage Point. New York, Academic Press, 1972
78. Risch N: Linkage strategies for genetically complex traits, I: multilocus models. Am J Hum Genet 1990; 46:222–228
79. Guttmacher AE, Collins FS: Genomic medicine—a primer. N Engl J Med 2002; 347:1512–1520
80. Maier W, Merikangas KR: Co-occurrence and cotransmission of affective disorders and alcoholism in families. Br J Psychiatry Suppl 1996; 168:93–100
81. Merikangas KR, Angst J, Eaton W, Canino G, Rubio-Stipec M, Wacker H, Wittchen HU, Andrade L, Essau C, Whitaker A, Kraemer H, Robins LN, Kupfer DJ: Comorbidity and boundaries of affective disorders with anxiety disorders and substance misuse: results of an international task force. Br J Psychiatry Suppl 1996; 30:58–67
82. Merikangas KR, Stevens DE, Fenton B, Stolar M, O'Malley S, Woods SW, Risch N: Comorbidity and familial aggregation of alcoholism and anxiety disorders. Psychol Med 1998; 28:773–788
83. Maier W, Lichtermann D, Minges J, Delmo C, Heun R: The relationship between bipolar disorder and alcoholism: a controlled family study. Psychol Med 1995; 25:787–796
84. Merikangas KR: Assortative mating for psychiatric disorders and psychological traits. Arch Gen Psychiatry 1982; 39:1173–1180
85. Galbaud du Fort G, Bland RC, Newman SC, Boothroyd LJ: Spouse similarity for lifetime psychiatric history in the general population. Psychol Med 1998; 28:789–802
86. Merikangas KR, Gelernter CS: Comorbidity for alcoholism and depression. Psychiatr Clin North Am 1990; 13:613–632
87. Merikangas KR, Rounsaville BJ, Prusoff BA: Familial factors in vulnerability to substance abuse, in Vulnerability to Drug Abuse. Edited by Glantz MD, Pickens RW. Washington, DC, American Psychological Association, 1992, pp 75–98
88. Kupfer DJ, First MB, Regier DA: A Research Agenda for DSM-V. Washington, DC, APA, 2002
89. Angst J, Merikangas KR, Preisig M: Subthreshold syndromes of depression and anxiety in the community. J Clin Psychiatry 1997; 58(suppl 8):6–10
90. Judd LL, Akiskal HS, Maser JD, Zeller PJ, Endicott J, Coryell W, Paulus MP, Kunovac JL, Leon AC, Mueller TI, Rice JA, Keller MB: A prospective 12-year study of subsyndromal and syndromal depressive symptoms in unipolar major depressive disorders. Arch Gen Psychiatry 1998; 55:694–700

91. Angst J, Merikangas KR: The depressive spectrum: diagnostic classification and course. J Affect Disord 1997; 45:31–40
92. Lenox RH, Gould TD, Manji HK: Endophenotypes in bipolar disorder. Am J Med Genet 2002; 114:391–406
93. Tsuang MT, Faraone SV, Lyons MJ: Identification of the phenotype in psychiatric genetics. Eur Arch Psychiatry Clin Neurosci 1993; 243:131–142
94. Faraone SV, Kremen WS, Lyons MJ, Pepple JR, Seidman LJ, Tsuang MT: Diagnostic accuracy and linkage analysis: how useful are schizophrenia spectrum phenotypes? Am J Psychiatry 1995; 152:1286–1290
95. Lichtermann D, Karbe E, Maier W: The genetic epidemiology of schizophrenia and of schizophrenia spectrum disorders. Eur Arch Psychiatry Clin Neurosci 2000; 250:304–310
96. Castellanos FX, Tannock R: Neuroscience of attention-deficit/hyperactivity disorder: the search for endophenotypes. Nat Rev Neurosci 2002; 3:617–628
97. Thompson PM, Rapoport JL, Cannon TD, Toga AW: Imaging the brain as schizophrenia develops: dynamic and genetic brain maps. Primary Psychiatry, Nov 2002, pp 40–44
98. Merikangas KR: Genetic epidemiology: bringing genetics to the population—the NAPE Lecture 2001. Acta Psychiatr Scand 2002; 105:3–13
99. Gordis L: Epidemiology. Philadelphia, WB Saunders, 2000
100. Ellsworth DL, Manolio TA: The emerging importance of genetics in epidemiologic research, II: issues in study design and gene mapping. Ann Epidemiol 1999; 9:75–90
101. Ellsworth DL, Manolio TA: The emerging importance of genetics in epidemiologic research, III: bioinformatics and statistical genetic methods. Ann Epidemiol 1999; 9:207–224
102. Khoury MJ, Beaty TH, Cohen BH: Fundamentals of Genetic Epidemiology. New York, Oxford University Press, 1993
103. Ödegaard Ö: Emigration and Insanity: A Study of Mental Disorders Among the Norwegian Born Population of Minnesota. Copenhagen, Levin & Munksgaards, 1932
104. Langholz B, Rothman N, Wacholder S, Thomas DC: Cohort studies for characterizing measured genes. J Natl Cancer Inst Monogr 1999; 26:39–42
105. Khoury MJ, Yang Q: The future of genetic studies of complex human disease: an epidemiologic perspective. Epidemiology 1998; 9:350–354
106. Thomas DC: Genetic epidemiology with a capital "E." Genet Epidemiol 2000; 19:289–300
107. Yang Q, Khoury MJ, Coughlin SC, Sun F, Flanders WD: On the use of population-based registries in the clinical validation of genetic tests for disease susceptibility. Genet Med 2000; 2:186–192
108. Khoury MJ, McCabe LL, McCabe ER: Population screening in the age of genomic medicine. N Engl J Med 2003; 348:50–58

109. Slooter A, van Duijn C: Genetic epidemiology of Alzheimer disease. Epidemiol Rev 1997; 19:107–119

110. Tol J, Roks G, Slooter AJ, van Duijn CM: Genetic and environmental factors in Alzheimer's disease. Rev Neurol (Paris) 1999; 155(suppl 4):S10–S16

111. Kivipelto M, Helkala EL, Laakso MP, Hanninen T, Hallikainen M, Alhainen K, Soininen H, Tuomilehto J, Nissinen A: Midlife vascular risk factors and Alzheimer's disease in later life: longitudinal, population based study. Br Med J 2001; 322:1447–1451

112. Munoz DG, Feldman H: Causes of Alzheimer's disease. Can Med Assoc J 2000; 162:65–72

113. Kivipelto M, Helkala EL, Laakso MP, Hanninen T, Hallikainen M, Alhainen K, Iivonen S, Mannermaa A, Tuomilehto J, Nissinen A, Soininen H: Apolipoprotein E epsilon 4 allele, elevated midlife total cholesterol level, and high midlife systolic blood pressure are independent risk factors for late-life Alzheimer disease. Ann Intern Med 2002; 137:149–155

114. Farrer LA, Cupples LA, Haines JL, Hyman B, Kukull WA, Mayeux R, Myers RH, Pericak-Vance MA, Risch N, van Duijn CM (APOE and Alzheimer Disease Meta Analysis Consortium): Effects of age, sex, and ethnicity on the association between apolipoprotein E genotype and Alzheimer disease: a meta-analysis. JAMA 1997; 278:1349–1356

115. Newman B, Millikan RC, King M: Genetic epidemiology of breast and ovarian cancers. Epidemiol Rev 1997; 19:69–79

116. Ottman R: An epidemiologic approach to gene-environment interaction. Genet Epidemiol 1990; 7:177–185

117. Smith PG, Day NE: The design of case-control studies: the influence of confounding and interaction effects. Int J Epidemiol 1984; 13:356–365

118. Hwang SJ, Beaty TH, Liang KY, Coresh J, Khoury MJ: Minimum sample size estimation to detect gene-environment interaction in case-control designs. Am J Epidemiol 1994; 140:1029–1037

119. Khoury MJ: Genetic epidemiology, in Modern Epidemiology, 2nd ed. Edited by Rothman K, Greenland S. Philadelphia, Lippincott-Raven, 1997

120. Yang Q, Khoury MJ: Evolving methods in genetic epidemiology, III: gene-environment interaction in epidemiologic research. Epidemiol Rev 1997; 19:33–43

121. Foppa I, Spiegelman D: Power and sample size calculations for case-control studies of gene-environment interactions with a polytomous exposure variable. Am J Epidemiol 1997; 146:596–604

122. Garcia-Closas M, Lubin JH: Power and sample size calculations in case-control studies of gene-environment interactions: comments on different approaches. Am J Epidemiol 1999; 149:689–692

123. Nebert DW, Ingelman-Sundberg M, Daly AK: Genetic epidemiology of environmental toxicity and cancer susceptibility: human allelic polymorphisms in drug-metabolizing enzyme genes, their functional importance, and nomenclature issues. Drug Metab Rev 1999; 31:467–487

124. Heath AC, Whitfield JB, Madden PA, Bucholz KK, Dinwiddie SH, Slutske WS, Bierut LJ, Statham DB, Martin NG: Towards a molecular epidemiology of alcohol dependence: analysing the interplay of genetic and environmental risk factors. Br J Psychiatry Suppl 2001; 40:S33–S40

125. Dick DM, Rose RJ, Viken RJ, Kaprio J, Koskenvuo M: Exploring gene-environment interactions: socioregional moderation of alcohol use. J Abnorm Psychol 2001; 110:625–632

126. Michael NL: Host genetic influences on HIV-1 pathogenesis. Curr Opin Immunol 1999; 11:466–474

127. Eaton WW, Addington AM, Bass J, Forman V, Gilbert S, Hayden K, Mielke M: Risk factors for major mental disorders: a review of the epidemiologic literature. Baltimore, Johns Hopkins University, Bloomberg School of Mental Health, Department of Mental Hygiene, Oct 2002. http://www.jhu.edu/~janthony/share/Envirome/Envirome-III-b.pdf

128. Gottesman II, Erlenmeyer-Kimling L: Family and twin strategies as a head start in defining prodromes and endophenotypes for hypothetical early interventions in schizophrenia. Schizophr Res 2001; 51:93–102

129. Meaney MJ: Maternal care, gene expression, and the transmission of individual differences in stress reactivity across generations. Annu Rev Neurosci 2001; 24:1161–1192

130. Varmus H: Getting ready for gene-based medicine. N Engl J Med 2002; 347:1526–1527

131. Hyman SE: The genetics of mental illness: implications for practice. Bull World Health Organ 2000; 78:455–463

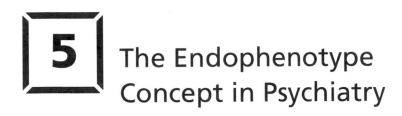

5 | The Endophenotype Concept in Psychiatry

Etymology and Strategic Intentions

Irving I. Gottesman, Ph.D., Hon. F.R.C.Psych.
Todd D. Gould, M.D.

As we celebrate the 50th anniversary of Nobelists Watson, Crick, and Wilkin's discovery (with Franklin) of the structure of DNA—and its offspring, the complete sequencing of the human genome—it is salutary to contemplate the relative youthfulness of the field of human genetics. The term "genetics" was provided by William Bateson in 1902 (the Wright brothers' first flight was in 1903). In 1909, the clarifying distinction we now take for granted between the concept of "genotype" and the concept of "phenotype" was provided by the Danish botanist Wilhelm Johanssen. He also introduced the word "gene." His research on self-fertilized lines of beans revealed that quantitative variability in the phenotype confounded thinking about separable contributions of heredity and environment. He found that the phenotype is often an imperfect indicator of the genotype, that the same genotype may give rise to a wide range of phenotypes, and that the same phenotype may have arisen from different genotypes. Specific evidence for multifactorial (genetic and nongenetic) contributions to a continuous phenotype was provided about the same time by

Dr. Gould is supported by the NIMH intramural research program.

The authors thank David A. Lewis, M.D., Husseini K. Manji, M.D., and Arturas Petronis, M.D., Ph.D., for their encouragement.

H. Nilsson-Ehle on the basis of observations of seed colors in crosses of oats and wheat. However, the term "polygene" was not available until K. Mather coined it in 1941. Exact citations for these historical references, often in German, are provided in the classic text by A.H. Sturtevant.[1]

Genotypes, which can be measured with techniques of molecular biology such as polymerase chain reaction (PCR) and DNA sequencing, are often useful as probabilistic prognosticators of disease. In contrast, a phenotype represents observable characteristics of an organism, which are the joint product of both genotypic *and* environmental influences. In diseases with classic or Mendelian genetics as their distal causes, genotypes are usually indicative of phenotypes. However, this degree of genetic certainty does not exist for diseases with complex genetics.[2–4] Genetic probabilism aptly describes the process by which a particular genotype gives rise to phenotype.[5, 6] Epigenetic factors may also be of critical importance for modifying the development of phenotypes,[7] and such modifications may be influenced by genotype or environment or be entirely stochastic in origin.[8] Thus, models of complex genetic disorders predict a ballet choreographed interactively over time among genotype, environment, and epigenetic factors, which gives rise to a particular phenotype.[9–12]

Despite the successful characterization of the nucleotide base-pair order that represents the human genome,[13, 14] and although a legion of genetic linkage and association studies have been done, psychiatry has had little success in definitively identifying "culprit" genes or gene regions in the development of diseases categorized by using the field's diagnostic classification schemas.[15–18] The reason there is so much difficulty is undoubtedly—in part—that psychiatry's classification systems describe heterogeneous disorders.[19–22] In addition to the inherent complexity of psychiatric diseases, which have multifactorial and polygenic origins, the brain is the most complex of all organs. In organs such as the liver, all cells are nearly identical in their phenotypes and very similar in their transcriptomes (mRNA transcripts) and proteomes. In addition to the homogeneity in the structure of such cells, their interactions are mostly homogeneous. However, individual cells of the brain are quite different from each other in their transcriptomes, proteomes, and morphological phenotypes and also in the thousands of connections and interactions with other neurons and glia that are critically important to optimal functioning. Different cellular experiences are transduced to differences on the biochemical and epigenetic levels so that cellular memories regulated by protein modification, morphometric changes, and epigenetic influences make the brain unique among organs. Furthermore, the brain is subject to complex interactions not just among genes, proteins, cells, and circuits of cells but also between individuals and their changing experiences.[23] Therefore, the phenotypic output from the brain, i.e., behavior, is not simply a sum of all its parts. It stands to reason that more optimally reduced measures of neuropsychiatric functioning should be more useful than behavioral "macros" in studies pursuing the biological and genetic components of psychiatric disorders.

The Endophenotype Concept in Psychiatry

The theory that genes and environment combine to confer susceptibility to the development of diseases surfaced in the early half of the last century, but the use of such a framework for exploring the etiology of schizophrenia and other psychiatric disorders is more recent. Douglas Falconer's 1965 multifactorial threshold model for diabetes and other common, non-Mendelizing diseases was adapted to a polygenic model of schizophrenia in 1967.[24] About this time, it became clear that the classification of psychiatric diseases on the basis of overt phenotypes (syndromic behaviors) might not be optimal for genetic dissection of these diseases, which have complex genetic underpinnings. In their writings summarizing genetic theories in schizophrenia 30 years ago, Gottesman and Shields[25, 26] described "endophenotypes" as internal phenotypes discoverable by a "biochemical test or microscopic examination." The term was adapted from a 1966 paper by John and Lewis,[27] who had used it to explain concepts in evolution and insect biology. They wrote that the geographical distribution of grasshoppers was a function of some feature not apparent in their "exophenotypes"; this feature was "the endophenotype, not the obvious and external but the microscopic and internal."

That felicitous term seemed to suit the needs of psychiatric genetics, and the concept of endophenotype was adapted for filling the gap between available descriptors and between the gene and the elusive disease processes. The identification of endophenotypes, which do not depend on what was obvious to the unaided eye, could help to resolve questions about etiological models. The rationale for the use of endophenotypes in exploring disease processes is illustrated in Figure 1. This rationale held that if the phenotypes associated with a disorder are very specialized and represent relatively straightforward and *putatively* more elementary phenomena (as opposed to behavioral macros), the number of genes required to produce variations in these traits may be

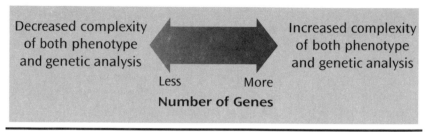

Figure 1.   Rationale for an endophenotype approach to genetic analysis of disorders with complex genetics

The number of genes involved in a phenotype is theorized to be directly related to both the complexity of the phenotype and the difficulty of genetic analysis.[28–34]

fewer than those involved in producing a psychiatric diagnostic entity. Endophenotypes provided a means for identifying the "downstream" traits or facets of clinical phenotypes, as well as the "upstream" consequences of genes and, in principle, could assist in the identification of aberrant genes in the hypothesized polygenic systems conferring vulnerabilities to disorders. That is, the intervening variables or hypothetical constructs that were championed as useful for theorizing about behaviors[35]—and that could mark the path between the genotype and the behavior of interest (Figure 2)—might Mendelize in a predicted manner.

Despite the inherent advantages of the concept of endophenotype, the term and its promise lay dormant for a number of years. However, now that multiple genetic linkage and association studies using current classification systems and the development of practical animal models, have all fallen short of success, the term and its usefulness have re-emerged. (A MEDLINE search for the years 2000 through 2002 found 62 entries for "endophenotype," compared with 16 entries before 2000.) Endophenotypes are being seen as a viable and perhaps necessary mechanism for overcoming the barriers to progress.[28, 51–58] The methods available for endophenotype analysis have advanced considerably since 1972; our current armamentarium includes neurophysiological, biochemical, endocrinological, neuroanatomical, cognitive, and neuropsychological (including configured self-report data) measures.[29] Advanced tools of neuroimaging such as functional magnetic resonance imaging (fMRI), morphometric MRI, diffusion tensor imaging, single photon emission computed tomography (SPECT), and positron emission tomography (PET) promise to expand the possibilities even more.[30, 59–61] Other terms with patently synonymous meaning, such as "intermediate phenotype," "biological marker," "subclinical trait," and

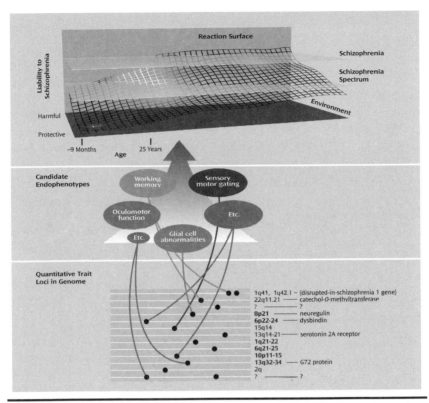

Figure 2. Gene regions, genes, and putative endophenotypes implicated in a biological systems approach to schizophrenia research
The reaction surface[36] suggests the dynamic developmental interplay among genetic, environmental, and epigenetic factors that produce cumulative liability to developing schizophrenia.[9–11, 37] Gene regions where linkage findings are more consistent are in bold, while gene regions corresponding to candidate genes or endophenotypes are shown in normal lettering.[16] Many of these endophenotypes are discussed in detailed reviews addressing overall strategies for schizophrenia discriminators,[38] sensory motor gating,[33, 39, 40] oculomotor function,[33, 40–43] working memory (sometimes synonymous with information processing, executive function, attention),[31, 32, 44–46] and glial cell abnormalities.[47] None of the sections of this figure can be definitive; many more gene loci, genes, and candidate endophenotypes exist and remain to be discovered (represented by question marks).[47, 48] Linkage and candidate gene studies have been the topic of recent reviews.[15, 16, 49, 50] The figure is not to scale. (Copyright 2003, I.I. Gottesman. Used with permission.)

"vulnerability marker," have been used interchangeably. These terms may not necessarily reflect genetic underpinnings but may rather reflect associated findings (see the discussion in the next section). In this context, we use the term "biological marker" to signify differences that do not have genetic underpinnings and "endophenotype" when certain heritability indicators are fulfilled.

Endophenotypes in Genetic Analysis

An endophenotype-based approach has the potential to assist in the genetic dissection of psychiatric diseases. Endophenotypes would ideally have monogenic roots; however, it is likely that many would have polygenic bases themselves. Furthermore, the use of endophenotypes in genetic research must be tempered by the realization that without controls and limits, their usefulness may be obscured. For example, putative endophenotypes do not necessarily reflect genetic effects. Indeed, these biological markers may be environmental, epigenetic, or multifactorial in origin. Criteria useful for the identification of markers in psychiatric genetics have been suggested[62] and have been adapted here to apply to endophenotypes:

1. The endophenotype is associated with illness in the population.
2. The endophenotype is heritable.
3. The endophenotype is primarily state-independent (manifests in an individual whether or not illness is active).
4. Within families, endophenotype and illness co-segregate.

    Subsequently, an additional criterion that may be useful for identifying endophenotypes of diseases that display complex inheritance patterns was suggested:[29]

5. The endophenotype found in affected family members is found in nonaffected family members at a higher rate than in the general population.

Other fields of medicine have had some success in using endophenotypes to assist with genetic linkage studies. For instance, the multiple genes that cause long QT syndrome were identified by using an endophenotype-based method.[63, 64] Manifestations of long QT syndrome include syncope, ventricle arrhythmias, and sudden death.[63] Although not all family members who carry the disease genes show these symptoms, a much greater percentage have QT elongation as measured by ECG. By using QT elongation as a phenotype—and excluding or including pedigree members with this finding—linkage studies were successful in identifying the genes that cause the QT elongation endophenotype and thus the syndrome phenotypes of syncope, ventricle arrhythmias, and sudden death.[64, 65] The identification of these genes has allowed for genetic manipulations in mice to study disease pathology and to further the development of novel medications.[66] Other examples in the literature of endophenotype-based strategies for identifying genetic linkage include studies of idiopathic hemochromatosis (excessive serum iron),[67] juvenile myoclonic epilepsy (an EEG abnormality),[68] and familial adenomatous polyposis coli (intestinal polyps).[69] In other disorders with complex genetics such as diabetes, hypercholesterolemia, or hypertension, researchers use physiological challenges, biochemical assays, and physiological measures to obtain a primary index of disease pathology. Indeed, these syndromes may all present to the physician as fatigue, but the pathophysiological underpinnings are substantially different. The glucose tolerance test, measurements of serum cholesterol levels, and sphygmomanometer measurements all represent objective, quantifiable methods for making disease diagnosis and classification. In addition to being crucial in diagnosis and classification of these diseases, the phenomena measured by these methods constitute endophenotypes that represent the *primary* inclusion/exclusion feature by which "hits" for genetic linkage and association studies are defined.

In psychiatry, a number of attempts have been made to develop and determine the feasibility of candidate endophenotypes. However, few have met all the criteria listed earlier. Nonetheless, some linkage and association studies—using endophenotypes—have had moderate success. Candidate endophenotypes have also been used in the development of animal models and to subtype patients for classification and diagnostic reasons (see the discussion in later sections). The hunt for candidate endophenotypes has been described in the literature on several psychiatric disorders, including schizophrenia,[30, 31–33, 39, 70–73] mood disorders,[28, 55, 74, 75] Alzheimer's disease,[76, 77] attention deficit hyperactivity disorder,[54, 78, 79] and even personality disorders.[80] We give a brief description of some possibilities in schizophrenia research as salient examples. The interested reader is referred to the references just cited for more in-depth discussions.

Sensory Motor Gating and Eye-Tracking Dysfunction in Schizophrenia

Deficits in sensory motor gating are consistent neuropsychological findings in schizophrenia.[33, 39] The hypothesized association between these deficits and schizophrenia has face validity primarily on the basis of patients' reports that they have difficulty filtering information from multiple sources.[33, 81–83] On the level of neurobiology, the inhibitory mechanisms of patients with schizophrenia may not be capable of adequately adjusting to the multiple distinct or repetitive inputs that occur in everyday life. Neuropsychological tests, including assessments of P50 suppression and prepulse inhibition of the startle response, have been developed to discern efficiencies in these capabilities. Both tasks have been studied in schizophrenic patients, and abnormalities consistent with defects in inhibitory neuronal circuits have been found.

In tests of prepulse inhibition, startling sensory stimuli (loud noise, bright light) are used to elicit an unconditional reflexive startle response in individuals. If a weaker prestimulus is provided before the startling stimulus, the subsequent startle response is generally diminished. A relatively reproducible finding is that this diminution of the second response is attenuated in patients with schizophrenia, compared to healthy subjects.[39, 84, 85] Prepulse inhibition is a generally conserved finding among vertebrates, and as such it has been the target of several rodent studies (reviewed in reference 86), both to model a facet of schizophrenia and to investigate the biology of a prepulse inhibition response. The presence of this candidate endophenotype has been documented in relatives of patients with schizophrenia,[87] but more extensive testing is required. Genetic studies in inbred animals have suggested at least a partial genetic diathesis;[86] however, environmental influences may also be active.[88, 89] Abnormal prepulse inhibition is not specific to schizophrenia; studies have identified this abnormality in obsessive-compulsive disorder[90] and Huntington's disease,[91] among others. However, the reproducibility of the finding in schizophrenia, the fact that abnormal prepulse inhibition parallels a putative central abnormality in the disease, and the fact that prepulse inhibition is a conserved phenomenon among vertebrates make abnormal prepulse inhibition a promising candidate endophenotype to pursue.

The P50 suppression test uses two auditory stimuli presented at 500-msec intervals. A positive event-related response for both stimuli is measured by EEG. In normal individuals, the neuronal response to the second stimulus is of lower amplitude than the first. However, patients with schizophrenia do not show the same degree of suppression of P50 amplitude.[33, 92–95] In addition to this finding in probands, abnormal P50 suppression is found in unaffected first-degree relatives of patients with schizophrenia.[95–99] The heritability of this measure has been assessed in twins, and the results have suggested that genetics plays a role in the development of variation in this candidate endophenotype.[100, 101] Freedman and colleagues[102] also used P50 suppression to identify a potential susceptibility locus for schizophrenia on chromosome 15, a chromosomal region where the gene for the $\alpha7$ nicotinic acetylcholine receptor resides. Furthermore, this group of researchers has shown linkage disequilibrium in this region[103] and has shown that promoter variants of the $\alpha7$ receptor are associated with schizophrenia and/or P50 suppression abnormalities.[104]

Eye-tracking dysfunction has long been associated with schizophrenia. This dysfunction was first described in 1908 by Diefendorf and Dodge,[105] whose work was rediscovered in the 1970s, initially by Holzman and colleagues.[106, 107]

Eye movements are generally of two forms, either saccadic (brief and extremely rapid movements) or smooth and controlled. The latter "smooth pursuit" eye movements occur only when the subject is following an object moving at a constant velocity, most commonly a pendulum (in early studies) or bright dot on a computer monitor. Initiation and maintenance of smooth pursuit eye movements involve integration of functions of the prefrontal cortex frontal eye fields, visual and vestibular circuitry, thalamus, and cerebellum, as well as the muscles and neural circuitry directly responsible for eye movement.[108]

A number of studies have found that patients with schizophrenia have deficiencies in smooth pursuit eye movements, compared to healthy subjects (see references 41–43 for review). In general, these deficiencies are manifested as corrective saccades, which follow smooth pursuit eye movements that are slightly slower than the target (reviewed in reference 42, where more detailed descriptions of specific abnormalities are available). Furthermore, the heritability of these deficiencies has been extensively addressed; studies have suggested that biological relatives of schizophrenic subjects have an increased rate of smooth pursuit eye movement dysfunction. Thus, 40%–80% of schizophrenic subjects, 25%–45% of their first-degree relatives, and less than 10% of healthy comparison subjects generally show this trait.[41–43] A study requiring replication has suggested linkage to a region of chromosome 6.[109] Correlating smooth pursuit function with neuroimaging measures[110] or performance on working memory tasks[111, 112] may be a useful research strategy. Smooth pursuit eye movements are maintained in primates but not in most other mammals used in preclinical research.[108]

Working Memory in Schizophrenia

Working memory and executive cognition are compromised in patients with schizophrenia.[44] A primary brain region involved in working memory is the dorsolateral prefrontal cortex,[31, 45, 113] a region in which abnormalities have been found in postmortem studies of schizophrenic patients.[114] Family,[115, 116] and twin studies[117, 118] have suggested heritability of working memory deficits in schizophrenia.

Recent studies have identified gene and chromosomal regions possibly involved in working memory. A study of Finnish twins by Gasperoni and colleagues,[53] which used an endophenotype-based strategy, suggested linkage and association to a region of chromosome 1. In their study, dizygotic twins discordant for schizophrenia underwent four neuropsychological tests. Using the sum of performance scores on these tests, Gasperoni and colleagues identified significant linkage to 1q41, a region previously suggested in traditional linkage studies of schizophrenia.[119–122] By stratifying their data according to performance on each neuropsychological test, they found that visual working memory performance was highly significantly linked with this region (p=0.007), while performance on none of the other three neuropsychological tests was significantly associated with any 1q markers. In the second part of their study, Gasperoni and colleagues[53] completed an association analysis involving monozygotic discordant twins, unaffected dizygotic and monozygotic twins, and the dizygotic twin group from the linkage study. In this analysis, an association of the 1q41 region and performance on the visual working memory task was again identified. The facts that previous linkage studies have identified this region *and* that performance on working memory tasks is a reproducible endophenotype for schizophrenia strengthen the claim that this endophenotype—and the putative gene(s) at 1q41 linked to it—may be relevant to the pathophysiology of schizophrenia. The study requires replication in a larger group of subjects representing a nonisolate population.

Association and physiological evidence have also linked a specific enzyme with a small increased risk for developing schizophrenia and with poorer performance on a working memory task. The enzyme catechol *O*-methyltransferase (COMT), the gene for which is found at 22q11.2, assists in the catabolism of dopamine. This chromosomal region has been linked to both schizophrenia and bipolar disorder and overlaps with a deletion that has been associated with velocardiofacial syndrome (DiGeorge syndrome) and schizophrenia (see reference 16 for review). A functional polymorphism (*val108/158met*) for COMT results in a fourfold increase in the activity of this enzyme. The considerable body of evidence implicating dopaminergic neurotransmission, the presence of a common functional polymorphism, and the data suggesting the involvement of the dorsolateral prefrontal cortex in schizophrenia and working memory led to association studies of COMT.[31]

While their effect sizes are small, a number of family studies have found that the valine allele is transmitted at a higher rate than the methionine allele to patients with schizophrenia than to their nonaffected siblings (reviewed in reference 31). This polymorphism has also been linked to performance on a working memory task. Specifically, Egan et al.[123] associated poorer performance on a working memory task in patients, their siblings, and comparison subjects with the same valine allele variation of COMT found to be transmitted at a higher rate in schizophrenia. They used fMRI to measure dorsolateral prefrontal cortex activation in a subset of these individuals; the fMRI fingerprint from individuals with the valine allele suggested that activation of the dorsolateral prefrontal cortex is less efficient in those subjects.[123] Additional studies from two independent laboratories have also suggested that patients with schizophrenia show this inefficiency.[124–126] Callicott and colleagues[127] have recently shown that the fMRI response in the dorsolateral prefrontal cortex observed in schizophrenic subjects is also found in unaffected siblings of patients with schizophrenia. Although they found no group differences between the siblings of schizophrenic patients and the comparison group in overall working memory performance, fMRI measurement showed that the sibling group had less efficient dorsolateral prefrontal cortex functioning than the comparison group. Taken together, these results suggest that fMRI analysis of subjects undergoing working memory tasks may be a more sensitive endophenotype than working memory performance alone as measured by neuropsychological testing. Additional studies using PET have suggested dysfunction of the cortical-thalamic-cerebellar-cortical circuit during working memory tasks.[72,73] The "cognitive dysmetria" resulting from this disruption may provide another candidate endophenotype.

Conclusion: Broader Uses for Endophenotypes

Endophenotypes may have additional uses in psychiatry, including uses in diagnosis, classification, and the development of animal models. The current classification schema in psychiatry were derived from observable clinical grounds to address the need for clinical description and communication.[22] However, they are not based on measures of the underlying genetic or biological pathophysiology of the disorders. The most widely used systems currently in place must serve the needs of clinicians, psychiatric statisticians, administrators, and insurance companies, among other groups and agencies.[128] As this system is designed for a wide range of users and because it pays little attention to the biological contributors to the disorders, it is not optimized for the design, implementation, and success of research studies.[128] The lack of a biological basis for the classification of psychiatric disorders has led, in part, to a lack of success in studies of the neurobiology and genetics of psychiatric disorders. Endophenotype-based analysis would be useful for establishing a biological underpinning for diagnosis and classification; a net outcome would be improved understanding of the neurobiology and genetics of psychopathology.

Animal models are an active area of research in psychiatry. However, despite some progress,[129, 130] there remains a great need for further development.[130–132] Improved animal models will help in understanding the neurobiology of psychiatric disorders and will further the development of truly novel medications.[133] Development of animal partial-models in psychiatry relies on identifying critical components of behavior (or other neurobiological traits) that are representative of more complex phenomena.[134] Animals will never have guilty ruminations, suicidal thoughts, or rapid speech. Thus, animal models based on endophenotypes that represent evolutionarily selected and quantifiable traits may better lend themselves to investigation of psychiatric phenomena than models based on face-valid diagnostic phenotypes.[28]

Given the hopefully successful consequences of studies adopting an endophenotype strategy, psychiatric diagnosis will continue to be important in research and clinical practice. Indeed, similar to the principle we describe here, optimally reduced or partitioned phenotypes may be useful in refining the diagnostic system. Measures that have already been used to deconstruct illnesses for genetic analysis include severity and course of illness,[135] age at onset of illness,[136, 137] amount of substance use in drug and alcohol disorders,[138, 139] and response to specific treatments such as lithium.[140, 141]

Gottesman and Shields[25] concluded their 1972 book on schizophrenia and genetics with the following remarks:

> We are optimistically hopeful that the current mass of research on families of schizophrenics will discover an endophenotype, either biological or behavioral (psychometric pattern), which will not only discriminate schizophrenics from other psychotics, but will also be found in all the identical co-twins of schizophrenics whether concordant or discordant. All genetic theorizing will benefit from the development of such an indicator. (p. 336)

Although these words are still pertinent after 30 years, there is ample reason to be optimistic about anticipated discoveries and refinements in the quest for endophenotypes.

References

1. Sturtevant AH: A History of Genetics. New York, Cold Spring Harbor Laboratory Press, 1965 (reprinted 2001) (full text available online at http://www.esp.org/books/sturt/history)
2. Zerba KE, Ferrell RE, Sing CF: Complex adaptive systems and human health: the influence of common genotypes of the apolipoprotein E (ApoE) gene polymorphism and age on the relational order within a field of lipid metabolism traits. Hum Genet 2000; 107:466–475
3. Sing CF, Zerba KE, Reilly SL: Traversing the biological complexity in the hierarchy between genome and CAD endpoints in the population at large. Clin Genet 1994; 46(1 special number):6–14
4. Province MA, Shannon WD, Rao DC: Classification methods for confronting heterogeneity. Adv Genet 2001; 42:273–286
5. Gottesman II: Psychopathology through a life span-genetic prism. Am Psychol 2001; 56:867–878
6. Merikangas KR, Swendsen JD: Genetic epidemiology of psychiatric disorders. Epidemiol Rev 1997; 19:144–155
7. Petronis A, Gottesman, II, Crow TJ, DeLisi LE, Klar AJ, Macciardi F, McInnis MG, McMahon FJ, Paterson AD, Skuse D, Sutherland GR: Psychiatric epigenetics: a new focus for the new century. Mol Psychiatry 2000; 5:342–346
8. Rakyan VK, Preis J, Morgan HD, Whitelaw E: The marks, mechanisms and memory of epigenetic states in mammals. Biochem J 2001; 356(part 1):1–10
9. McGuffin P, Owen MJ, Gottesman II: Psychiatric Genetics and Genomics. Oxford, UK, Oxford University Press, 2002
10. Lewis DA, Levitt P: Schizophrenia as a disorder of neurodevelopment. Annu Rev Neurosci 2002; 25:409–432
11. Petronis A: Human morbid genetics revisited: relevance of epigenetics. Trends Genet 2001; 17:142–146
12. Glazier AM, Nadeau JH, Aitman TJ: Finding genes that underlie complex traits. Science 2002; 298:2345–2349
13. Venter JC, Adams MD, Myers EW, Li PW, Mural RJ, Sutton GG, Smith HO, Yandell M, Evans CA, Holt RA, Gocayne JD, Amanatides P, et al: The sequence of the human genome. Science 2001; 291:1304–1305; correction, 2001; 292:1838
14. Lander ES, Linton LM, Birren B, Nusbaum C, Zody MC, Baldwin J, Devon K, Dewar K, Doyle M, FitzHugh W, Funke R, Gage D, et al: Initial sequencing and analysis of the human genome. Nature 2001; 409:860–921
15. Cowan WM, Kopnisky KL, Hyman SE: The human genome project and its impact on psychiatry. Annu Rev Neurosci 2002; 25:1–50
16. Sklar P: Linkage analysis in psychiatric disorders: the emerging picture. Annu Rev Genomics Hum Genet 2002; 3:371–413

17. Gottesman II, Moldin SO: Schizophrenia genetics at the millennium: cautious optimism. Clin Genet 1997; 52:404–407

18. Cloninger CR: The discovery of susceptibility genes for mental disorders. Proc Natl Acad Sci USA 2002; 99:13365–13367

19. Andreasen NC: Understanding the causes of schizophrenia (letter). N Engl J Med 1999; 340:645–647

20. Lewis DA: In pursuit of the pathogenesis and pathophysiology of schizophrenia: where do we stand? (editorial). Am J Psychiatry 2002; 159:1467–1469

21. Chakravarti A, Little P: Nature, nurture and human disease. Nature 2003; 421:412–414

22. Andreasen NC: Schizophrenia: the fundamental questions. Brain Res Brain Res Rev 2000; 31:106–112

23. Kandel ER: A new intellectual framework for psychiatry. Am J Psychiatry 1998; 155:457–469

24. Gottesman, II, Shields J: A polygenic theory of schizophrenia. Proc Natl Acad Sci USA 1967; 58:199–205

25. Gottesman II, Shields J: Schizophrenia and Genetics: A Twin Study Vantage Point. New York, Academic Press, 1972

26. Gottesman II, Shields J: Genetic theorizing and schizophrenia. Br J Psychiatry 1973; 122:15–30

27. John B, Lewis KR: Chromosome variability and geographical distribution in insects: chromosome rather than gene variation provide the key to differences among populations. Science 1966; 152:711–721

28. Lenox RH, Gould TD, Manji HK: Endophenotypes in bipolar disorder. Am J Med Genet 2002; 114:391–406

29. Leboyer M, Bellivier F, Nosten-Bertrand M, Jouvent R, Pauls D, Mallet J: Psychiatric genetics: search for phenotypes. Trends Neurosci 1998; 21:102–105

30. Callicott JH, Weinberger DR: Brain imaging as an approach to phenotype characterization for genetic studies of schizophrenia. Methods Mol Med 2003; 77:227–247

31. Weinberger DR, Egan MF, Bertolino A, Callicott JH, Mattay VS, Lipska BK, Berman KF, Goldberg TE: Prefrontal neurons and the genetics of schizophrenia. Biol Psychiatry 2001; 50:825–844

32. Egan MF, Goldberg TE: Intermediate cognitive phenotypes associated with schizophrenia. Methods Mol Med 2003; 77:163–197

33. Braff DL, Freedman R: Endophenotypes in studies of the genetics of schizophrenia, in Neuropsychopharmacology: The Fifth Generation of Progress. Edited by Davis KL, Charney DS, Coyle JT, Nemeroff C. Philadelphia, Lippincott Williams & Wilkins, 2002, pp 703–716

34. Leboyer M: Searching for alternative phenotypes in psychiatric genetics. Methods Mol Med 2003; 77:145–161

35. MacCorquodale K, Meehl PE: On a distinction between hypothetical constructs and intervening variables. Psychol Rev 1948; 55:95–107

36. Turkheimer E, Goldsmith HH, Gottesman II: Commentary: some conceptual deficiencies in "developmental" behavior genetics. Hum Dev 1995; 38:142–153

37. Faraone SV, Tsuang D, Tsuang MT: Genetics of Mental Disorders: A Guide for Students, Clinicians, and Researchers. New York, Guilford, 1999

38. Heinrichs RW: In Search of Madness: Schizophrenia and Neuroscience. New York, Oxford University Press, 2001

39. Braff DL, Geyer MA, Swerdlow NR: Human studies of prepulse inhibition of startle: normal subjects, patient groups, and pharmacological studies. Psychopharmacology (Berl) 2001; 156:234–258

40. Freedman R: Electrophysiological phenotypes. Methods Mol Med 2003; 77:215–225

41. Holzman PS: Less is truly more: psychopathology research in the 21st century, in Principles of Psychopathology: Essays in Honor of Brendan A. Maher. Edited by Lenzenweger MF, Hooley JM. Washington, American Psychological Association, 2003, pp 175–194

42. Calkins ME, Iacono WG: Eye movement dysfunction in schizophrenia: a heritable characteristic for enhancing phenotype definition. Am J Med Genet 2000; 97:72–76

43. Lee KH, Williams LM: Eye movement dysfunction as a biological marker of risk for schizophrenia. Aust N Z J Psychiatry 2000; 34(Suppl):S91–S100

44. Goldberg TE, Green MF: Neurocognitive functioning in patients with schizophrenia: an overview, in Neuropsychopharmacology: The Fifth Generation of Progress. Edited by Davis KL, Charney DS, Coyle JT, Nemeroff C. Philadelphia, Lippincott Williams & Wilkins, 2002, pp 657–669

45. Goldman-Rakic PS: The physiological approach: functional architecture of working memory and disordered cognition in schizophrenia. Biol Psychiatry 1999; 46:650–661

46. Erlenmeyer-Kimling L, Rock D, Roberts SA, Janal M, Kestenbaum C, Cornblatt B, Adamo UH, Gottesman II: Attention, memory, and motor skills as childhood predictors of schizophrenia-related psychoses: the New York High-Risk Project. Am J Psychiatry 2000; 157:1416–1422

47. Moises HW, Zoega T, Gottesman II: The glial growth factors deficiency and synaptic destabilization hypothesis of schizophrenia. BMC Psychiatry 2002; 2:8, http://www.biomedcentral.com/1471-244X/2/8/

48. Wise LH, Lanchbury JS, Lewis CM: Meta-analysis of genome searches. Ann Hum Genet 1999; 63(part 3):263–272

49. Owen MJ, O'Donovan MC, Gottesman II: Schizophrenia, in Psychiatric Genetics and Genomics. Edited by McGuffin P, Owens MJ, Gottesman II. Oxford, UK, Oxford University Press, 2002, pp 247–266

50. Pulver AE, Pearlson G, McGrath J, Lasseter VK, Swarts K, Papadimitriou G: Schizophrenia, in The Genetic Basis of Common Diseases. Edited by King RA, Rotter JI, Motulsky AG. New York, Oxford University Press, 2002

51. Trumbetta SL, Gottesman II: Endophenotypes for marital status in the NAS-NRC Twin Registry, in Genetic Influences on Human Fertility and Sexuality. Edited by Rodgers JL, Rowe DC, Miller WB. Boston, Kluwer Academic, 2000, pp 253–269

52. Skuse DH: Endophenotypes and child psychiatry. Br J Psychiatry 2001; 178:395–396

53. Gasperoni TL, Ekelund J, Huttunen M, Palmer CG, Tuulio-Henriksson A, Lonnqvist J, Kaprio J, Peltonen L, Cannon TD: Genetic linkage and association between chromosome 1q and working memory function in schizophrenia. Am J Med Genet 2003; 116(1 suppl):8–16

54. Castellanos FX, Tannock R: Neuroscience of attention-deficit/hyperactivity disorder: the search for endophenotypes. Nat Rev Neurosci 2002; 3:617–628

55. Ahearn EP, Speer MC, Chen YT, Steffens DC, Cassidy F, Van Meter S, Provenzale JM, Weisler RH, Krishnan KR: Investigation of Notch3 as a candidate gene for bipolar disorder using brain hyperintensities as an endophenotype. Am J Med Genet 2002; 114:652–658

56. Cadenhead KS, Light GA, Geyer MA, McDowell JE, Braff DL: Neurobiological measures of schizotypal personality disorder: defining an inhibitory endophenotype? Am J Psychiatry 2002; 159:869–871

57. Cornblatt BA, Malhotra AK: Impaired attention as an endophenotype for molecular genetic studies of schizophrenia. Am J Med Genet 2001; 105:11–15

58. Merikangas KR, Chakravarti A, Moldin SO, Araj H, Blangero JC, Burmeister M, Crabbe J Jr, Depaulo JR Jr, Foulks E, Freimer NB, Koretz DS, Lichtenstein W, Mignot E, Reiss AL, Risch NJ, Takahashi JS: Future of genetics of mood disorders research. Biol Psychiatry 2002; 52:457–477

59. Seibyl JP, Scanley E, Krystal JH, Innis RB: Neuroimaging methodologies, in Neurobiology of Mental Illness. Edited by Charney DS, Nester EJ, Bunney BS. New York, Oxford University Press, 1999, pp 170–189

60. Diwadkar VA, Keshavan MS: Newer techniques in magnetic resonance imaging and their potential for neuropsychiatric research. J Psychosom Res 2002; 53:677–685

61. Martinez D, Broft A, Laruelle M: Imaging neurochemical endophenotypes: promises and pitfalls. Pharmacogenomics 2001; 2:223–237

62. Gershon ES, Goldin LR: Clinical methods in psychiatric genetics, I: robustness of genetic marker investigative strategies. Acta Psychiatr Scand 1986; 74:113–118

63. Keating MT, Sanguinetti MC: Molecular and cellular mechanisms of cardiac arrhythmias. Cell 2001; 104:569–580

64. Keating M, Atkinson D, Dunn C, Timothy K, Vincent GM, Leppert M: Linkage of a cardiac arrhythmia, the long QT syndrome, and the Harvey ras-1 gene. Science 1991; 252:704–706

65. Vincent GM, Timothy KW, Leppert M, Keating M: The spectrum of symptoms and QT intervals in carriers of the gene for the long-QT syndrome. N Engl J Med 1992; 327:846–852

66. Casimiro MC, Knollmann BC, Ebert SN, Vary JC Jr, Greene AE, Franz MR, Grinberg A, Huang SP, Pfeifer K: Targeted disruption of the Kcnq1 gene produces a mouse model of Jervell and Lange-Nielsen syndrome. Proc Natl Acad Sci USA 2001; 98:2526–2531

67. Lalouel JM, Le Mignon L, Simon M, Fauchet R, Bourel M, Rao DC, Morton NE: Genetic analysis of idiopathic hemochromatosis using both qualitative (disease status) and quantitative (serum iron) information. Am J Hum Genet 1985; 37:700–718

68. Greenberg DA, Delgado-Escueta AV, Widelitz H, Sparkes RS, Treiman L, Maldonado HM, Park MS, Terasaki PI: Juvenile myoclonic epilepsy (JME) may be linked to the BF and HLA loci on human chromosome 6. Am J Med Genet 1988; 31:185–192

69. Leppert M, Burt R, Hughes JP, Samowitz W, Nakamura Y, Woodward S, Gardner E, Lalouel JM, White R: Genetic analysis of an inherited predisposition to colon cancer in a family with a variable number of adenomatous polyps. N Engl J Med 1990; 322:904–908

70. Gottesman II, Erlenmeyer-Kimling L: Family and twin strategies as a head start in defining prodromes and endophenotypes for hypothetical early-interventions in schizophrenia. Schizophr Res 2001; 51:93–102

71. Lenzenweger MF: Schizophrenia: refining the phenotype, resolving endophenotypes. Behav Res Ther 1999; 37:281–295

72. Andreasen NC, O'Leary DS, Cizadlo T, Arndt S, Rezai K, Ponto LL, Watkins GL, Hichwa RD: Schizophrenia and cognitive dysmetria: a positron-emission tomography study of dysfunctional prefrontal-thalamic-cerebellar circuitry. Proc Natl Acad Sci U S A 1996; 93:9985–9990

73. Andreasen NC, Nopoulos P, O'Leary DS, Miller DD, Wassink T, Flaum M: Defining the phenotype of schizophrenia: cognitive dysmetria and its neural mechanisms. Biol Psychiatry 1999; 46:908–920

74. Berman RM, Narasimhan M, Miller HL, Anand A, Cappiello A, Oren DA, Heninger GR, Charney DS: Transient depressive relapse induced by catecholamine depletion: potential phenotypic vulnerability marker? Arch Gen Psychiatry 1999; 56:395–403

75. Niculescu AB III, Akiskal HS: Proposed endophenotypes of dysthymia: evolutionary, clinical and pharmacogenomic considerations. Mol Psychiatry 2001; 6:363–366

76. Neugroschl J, Davis KL: Biological markers in Alzheimer disease. Am J Geriatr Psychiatry 2002; 10:660–677

77. Kurz A, Riemenschneider M, Drzezga A, Lautenschlager N: The role of biological markers in the early and differential diagnosis of Alzheimer's disease. J Neural Transm Suppl 2002:127–133

78. Gould TD, Bastain TM, Israel ME, Hommer DW, Castellanos FX: Altered performance on an ocular fixation task in attention-deficit/hyperactivity disorder. Biol Psychiatry 2001; 50:633–635

79. Seidman LJ, Biederman J, Monuteaux MC, Weber W, Faraone SV: Neuropsychological functioning in nonreferred siblings of children with attention deficit/hyperactivity disorder. J Abnorm Psychol 2000; 109:252–265

80. New AS, Siever LJ: Biochemical endophenotypes in personality disorders. Methods Mol Med 2003; 77:199–213

81. Braff DL, Geyer MA: Sensorimotor gating and schizophrenia: human and animal model studies. Arch Gen Psychiatry 1990; 47:181–188

82. Grillon C, Courchesne E, Ameli R, Geyer MA, Braff DL: Increased distractibility in schizophrenic patients: electrophysiologic and behavioral evidence. Arch Gen Psychiatry 1990; 47:171–179

83. McGhie A, Chapman J: Disorders of attention and perception in early schizophrenia. Br J Med Psychol 1961; 34:103–116

84. Braff DL: Psychophysiological and information-processing approaches to schizophrenia, in Neurobiology of Mental Illness. Edited by Charney DS, Nester EJ, Bunney BS. New York, Oxford University Press, 1999, pp 258–271

85. Braff DL, Grillon C, Geyer MA: Gating and habituation of the startle reflex in schizophrenic patients. Arch Gen Psychiatry 1992; 49:206–215

86. Geyer MA, McIlwain KL, Paylor R: Mouse genetic models for prepulse inhibition: an early review. Mol Psychiatry 2002; 7:1039–1053

87. Cadenhead KS, Swerdlow NR, Shafer KM, Diaz M, Braff DL: Modulation of the startle response and startle laterality in relatives of schizophrenic patients and in subjects with schizotypal personality disorder: evidence of inhibitory deficits. Am J Psychiatry 2000; 157:1660–1668; correction, 157:1904

88. Ellenbroek BA, Cools AR: Early maternal deprivation and prepulse inhibition: the role of the postdeprivation environment. Pharmacol Biochem Behav 2002; 73:177–184

89. Weiss IC, Feldon J: Environmental animal models for sensorimotor gating deficiencies in schizophrenia: a review. Psychopharmacology (Berl) 2001; 156:305–326

90. Swerdlow NR, Benbow CH, Zisook S, Geyer MA, Braff DL: A preliminary assessment of sensorimotor gating in patients with obsessive compulsive disorder. Biol Psychiatry 1993; 33:298–301

91. Swerdlow NR, Paulsen J, Braff DL, Butters N, Geyer MA, Swenson MR: Impaired prepulse inhibition of acoustic and tactile startle response in patients with Huntington's disease. J Neurol Neurosurg Psychiatry 1995; 58:192–200

92. Adler LE, Pachtman E, Franks RD, Pecevich M, Waldo MC, Freedman R: Neurophysiological evidence for a defect in neuronal mechanisms involved in sensory gating in schizophrenia. Biol Psychiatry 1982; 17:639–654

93. Freedman R, Adler LE, Waldo MC, Pachtman E, Franks RD: Neurophysiological evidence for a defect in inhibitory pathways in schizophrenia: comparison of medicated and drug-free patients. Biol Psychiatry 1983; 18:537–551

94. Freedman R, Adler LE, Gerhardt GA, Waldo M, Baker N, Rose GM, Drebing C, Nagamoto H, Bickford-Wimer P, Franks R: Neurobiological studies of sensory gating in schizophrenia. Schizophr Bull 1987; 13:669–678

95. Siegel C, Waldo M, Mizner G, Adler LE, Freedman R: Deficits in sensory gating in schizophrenic patients and their relatives: evidence obtained with auditory evoked responses. Arch Gen Psychiatry 1984; 41:607–612

96. Myles-Worsley M: P50 sensory gating in multiplex schizophrenia families from a Pacific Island isolate. Am J Psychiatry 2002; 159:2007–2012

97. Clementz BA, Geyer MA, Braff DL: Poor P50 suppression among schizophrenia patients and their first-degree biological relatives. Am J Psychiatry 1998; 155:1691–1694

98. Waldo MC, Carey G, Myles-Worsley M, Cawthra E, Adler LE, Nagamoto HT, Wender P, Byerley W, Plaetke R, Freedman R: Codistribution of a sensory gating deficit and schizophrenia in multi-affected families. Psychiatry Res 1991; 39:257–268

99. Waldo M, Myles-Worsley M, Madison A, Byerley W, Freedman R: Sensory gating deficits in parents of schizophrenics. Am J Med Genet 1995; 60:506–511

100. Myles-Worsley M, Coon H, Byerley W, Waldo M, Young D, Freedman R: Developmental and genetic influences on the P50 sensory gating phenotype. Biol Psychiatry 1996; 39:289–295

101. Young DA, Waldo M, Rutledge JH III, Freedman R: Heritability of inhibitory gating of the P50 auditory-evoked potential in monozygotic and dizygotic twins. Neuropsychobiology 1996; 33:113–117

102. Freedman R, Coon H, Myles-Worsley M, Orr-Urtreger A, Olincy A, Davis A, Polymeropoulos M, Holik J, Hopkins J, Hoff M, Rosenthal J, Waldo MC, Reimherr F, Wender P, Yaw J, Young DA, Breese CR, Adams C, Patterson D, Adler LE, Kruglyak L, Leonard S, Byerley W: Linkage of a neurophysiological deficit in schizophrenia to a chromosome 15 locus. Proc Natl Acad Sci USA 1997; 94:587–592

103. Freedman R, Leonard S, Gault JM, Hopkins J, Cloninger CR, Kaufmann CA, Tsuang MT, Faraone SV, Malaspina D, Svrakic DM, Sanders A, Gejman P: Linkage disequilibrium for schizophrenia at the chromosome 15q13-14 locus of the α7-nicotinic acetylcholine receptor subunit gene (CHRNA7). Am J Med Genet 2001; 105:20–22

104. Leonard S, Gault J, Hopkins J, Logel J, Vianzon R, Short M, Drebing C, Berger R, Venn D, Sirota P, Zerbe G, Olincy A, Ross RG, Adler LE, Freedman R: Association of promoter variants in the α7 nicotinic acetylcholine receptor subunit gene with an inhibitory deficit found in schizophrenia. Arch Gen Psychiatry 2002; 59:1085–1096

105. Diefendorf AR, Dodge R: An experimental study of the ocular reactions of the insane from photographic records. Brain 1908; 31:451–489

106. Holzman PS, Proctor LR, Hughes DW: Eye-tracking patterns in schizophrenia. Science 1973; 181:179–181

107. Holzman PS, Proctor LR, Levy DL, Yasillo NJ, Meltzer HY, Hurt SW: Eye-tracking dysfunctions in schizophrenic patients and their relatives. Arch Gen Psychiatry 1974; 31:143–151

108. Munoz DP: Commentary: saccadic eye movements: overview of neural circuitry. Prog Brain Res 2002; 140:89–96

109. Arolt V, Lencer R, Nolte A, Muller-Myhsok B, Purmann S, Schurmann M, Leutelt J, Pinnow M, Schwinger E: Eye tracking dysfunction is a putative phenotypic susceptibility marker of schizophrenia and maps to a locus on chromosome 6p in families with multiple occurrence of the disease. Am J Med Genet 1996; 67(6):564–579

110. O'Driscoll GA, Benkelfat C, Florencio PS, Wolff AL, Joober R, Lal S, Evans AC: Neural correlates of eye tracking deficits in first-degree relatives of schizophrenic patients: a positron emission tomography study. Arch Gen Psychiatry 1999; 56:1127–1134

111. Park S, Lee J: Spatial working memory function in schizophrenia, in Principles of Psychopathology: Essays in Honor of Brendan A. Maher. Edited by Lenzenweger MF, Hooley JM. Washington, American Psychological Association, 2003, pp 83–106

112. Snitz BE, Curtis CE, Zald DH, Katsanis J, Iacono WG: Neuropsychological and oculomotor correlates of spatial working memory performance in schizophrenia patients and controls. Schizophr Res 1999; 38(1):37–50

113. Levy R, Goldman-Rakic PS: Segregation of working memory functions within the dorsolateral prefrontal cortex. Exp Brain Res 2000; 133:23–32

114. Harrison PJ: The neuropathology of schizophrenia: a critical review of the data and their interpretation. Brain 1999; 122(part 4):593–624

115. Park S, Holzman PS, Goldman-Rakic PS: Spatial working memory deficits in the relatives of schizophrenic patients. Arch Gen Psychiatry 1995; 52:821–828

116. Conklin HM, Curtis CE, Katsanis J, Iacono WG: Verbal working memory impairment in schizophrenia patients and their first-degree relatives: evidence from the Digit Span Task. Am J Psychiatry 2000; 157:275–277

117. Cannon TD, Huttunen MO, Lonnqvist J, Tuulio-Henriksson A, Pirkola T, Glahn D, Finkelstein J, Hietanen M, Kaprio J, Koskenvuo M: The inheritance of neuropsychological dysfunction in twins discordant for schizophrenia. Am J Hum Genet 2000; 67:369–382

118. Goldberg TE, Kelsoe JR, Weinberger DR, Pliskin NH, Kirwin PD, Berman KF: Performance of schizophrenic patients on putative neuropsychological tests of frontal lobe function. Int J Neurosci 1988; 42:51–58

119. Hovatta I, Varilo T, Suvisaari J, Terwilliger JD, Ollikainen V, Arajarvi R, Juvonen H, Kokko-Sahin ML, Vaisanen L, Mannila H, Lonnqvist J, Peltonen L: A genomewide screen for schizophrenia genes in an isolated Finnish subpopulation, suggesting multiple susceptibility loci. Am J Hum Genet 1999; 65:1114–1124

120. Ekelund J, Lichtermann D, Hovatta I, Ellonen P, Suvisaari J, Terwilliger JD, Juvonen H, Varilo T, Arajarvi R, Kokko-Sahin ML, Lonnqvist J, Peltonen L: Genome-wide scan for schizophrenia in the Finnish population: evidence for a locus on chromosome 7q22. Hum Mol Genet 2000; 9:1049–1057

121. St Clair D, Blackwood D, Muir W, Carothers A, Walker M, Spowart G, Gosden C, Evans HJ: Association within a family of a balanced autosomal translocation with major mental illness. Lancet 1990; 336:13–16

122. Millar JK, Wilson-Annan JC, Anderson S, Christie S, Taylor MS, Semple CA, Devon RS, Clair DM, Muir WJ, Blackwood DH, Porteous DJ: Disruption of two novel genes by a translocation co-segregating with schizophrenia. Hum Mol Genet 2000; 9:1415–1423

123. Egan MF, Goldberg TE, Kolachana BS, Callicott JH, Mazzanti CM, Straub RE, Goldman D, Weinberger DR: Effect of COMT Val108/158 Met genotype on frontal lobe function and risk for schizophrenia. Proc Natl Acad Sci USA 2001; 98:6917–6922

124. Manoach DS, Gollub RL, Benson ES, Searl MM, Goff DC, Halpern E, Saper CB, Rauch SL: Schizophrenic subjects show aberrant fMRI activation of dorsolateral prefrontal cortex and basal ganglia during working memory performance. Biol Psychiatry 2000; 48:99–109

125. Manoach DS, Press DZ, Thangaraj V, Searl MM, Goff DC, Halpern E, Saper CB, Warach S: Schizophrenic subjects activate dorsolateral prefrontal cortex during a working memory task, as measured by fMRI. Biol Psychiatry 1999; 45:1128–1137

126. Callicott JH, Bertolino A, Mattay VS, Langheim FJ, Duyn J, Coppola R, Goldberg TE, Weinberger DR: Physiological dysfunction of the dorsolateral prefrontal cortex in schizophrenia revisited. Cereb Cortex 2000; 10:1078–1092

127. Callicott JH, Egan MF, Mattay VS, Bertolino A, Bone AD, Verchinksi B, Weinberger DR: Abnormal fMRI response of the dorsolateral prefrontal cortex in cognitively intact siblings of patients with schizophrenia. Am J Psychiatry 2003; 160:709–719

128. Duffy A, Grof P: Psychiatric diagnoses in the context of genetic studies of bipolar disorder. Bipolar Disord 2001; 3:270–275

129. Crawley JN: What's Wrong With My Mouse? Behavioral Phenotyping of Transgenic and Knockout Mice. New York, Wiley-Liss, 2000

130. Einat H, Belmaker RH, Manji HK: New approaches to modeling bipolar disorder. Psychopharmacol Bull (in press)

131. Nestler EJ, Gould E, Manji H, Buncan M, Duman RS, Greshenfeld HK, Hen R, Koester S, Lederhendler I, Meaney M, Robbins T, Winsky L, Zalcman S: Preclinical models: status of basic research in depression. Biol Psychiatry 2002; 52:503–528

132. Einat H, Kofman O, Belmaker RH: Animal models of bipolar disorder: from a single episode to progressive cycling models, in Contemporary Issues in Modeling Psychopharmacology. Edited by Weiner I. Boston, Kluwer Academic, 2000, pp 165–180

133. Gould TD, Gray NA, Manji HK: The cellular neurobiology of severe mood and anxiety disorders: implications for the development of novel therapeutics, in Molecular Neurobiology for the Clinician. Edited by Charney DS. Washington, American Psychiatric Publishing (in press)

134. Crawley JN: Behavioral phenotyping of transgenic and knockout mice: experimental design and evaluation of general health, sensory functions, motor abilities, and specific behavioral tests. Brain Res 1999; 835:18–26

135. Geller B, Cook EH Jr: Ultradian rapid cycling in prepubertal and early adolescent bipolarity is not in transmission disequilibrium with val/met COMT alleles. Biol Psychiatry 2000; 47:605–609

136. Cardno AG, Holmans PA, Rees MI, Jones LA, McCarthy GM, Hamshere ML, Williams NM, Norton N, Williams HJ, Fenton I, Murphy KC, Sanders RD, Gray MY, O'Donovan MC, McGuffin P, Owen MJ: A genomewide linkage study of age at onset in schizophrenia. Am J Med Genet 2001; 105:439–445

137. Zubenko GS, Hughes HB, Stiffler JS, Zubenko WN, Kaplan BB: Genome survey for susceptibility loci for recurrent, early-onset major depression: results at 10cM resolution. Am J Med Genet 2002; 114:413–422

138. Wall TL, Carr LG, Ehlers CL: Protective association of genetic variation in alcohol dehydrogenase with alcohol dependence in Native American Mission Indians. Am J Psychiatry 2003; 160:41–46

139. Saccone NL, Kwon JM, Corbett J, Goate A, Rochberg N, Edenberg HJ, Foroud T, Li TK, Begleiter H, Reich T, Rice JP: A genome screen of maximum number of drinks as an alcoholism phenotype. Am J Med Genet 2000; 96:632–637

140. Mansour HA, Alda M, Nimgaonkar VL: Pharmacogenetics of bipolar disorder. Curr Psychiatry Rep 2002; 4:117–123

141. Detera-Wadleigh SD: Lithium-related genetics of bipolar disorder. Ann Med 2001; 33:272–285

6

The Genes and Brains of Mice and Men

Laurence H. Tecott, M.D., Ph.D.

The elucidation of the human genome will profoundly impact our understanding of human biology. This remarkable achievement enables the identification of the full complement of approximately 30,000 human genes, and it permits new insights into the pathophysiology and treatment of disease. However, genes cannot be systematically manipulated in humans, so we must therefore turn to other organisms to investigate gene function. In recognition of the importance of the mouse as the organism of choice for investigating gene function in the context of mammalian biology, the National Institutes of Health convened a scientific panel that recommended the generation of a "working draft" sequence of the mouse genome by 2003. This deadline was recently met by an international Mouse Genome Sequencing Consortium[1, 2]—an accomplishment that has been heralded as a development of major importance and a boon to investigators working in many areas of biomedical research.[3, 4] With the mouse genome sequence in hand, and a formidable array of molecular genetic technologies permitting its manipulation, unprecedented opportunities currently exist to apply these advances to the study of brain function and the physiological underpinnings of psychiatric disorders.

Supported by NIMH Independent Scientist Award MH-01949 and a National Alliance for Research on Schizophrenia and Depression Independent Investigator Award.

The author thanks Adele Dorison, Teresa McGuinness, Andrew Peterson, Samuel Barondes, Steven Hamilton, and Paul Ekman for helpful comments.

The Ascent of the Mouse

A number of practical and historical considerations have contributed to a rapid escalation in the use of mice for biomedical research. As fellow mammals, mice and humans possess similar body plans, organ systems, and mechanisms of physiological regulation. Comparative genomic analyses indicate that the divergence of mammalian lineages giving rise to humans and mice occurred approximately 75 million years ago, a relatively recent event by evolutionary standards.[5, 6] The genomes of humans and mice are approximately 2.9 and 2.5 billion nucleotides long, respectively, and both encode approximately 30,000 genes.[2] Approximately 99% of mouse genes have human counterparts—conversely, mouse versions (orthologs) can be identified for 99% of human genes. Furthermore, a large proportion of the mouse and human genomes are "syntenic," i.e., they possess chromosomal regions with the same order of genes. Approximately 96% of mouse genes are found in such syntenic regions. The high level of genomic homology between these species lends support to the view that what distinguishes humans from other mammals relates more to differences in how their genes are regulated and processed than to differences in the identities or numbers of the genes themselves.[7, 8]

Historically, the potential benefits of mice have not always been widely appreciated, as reflected by the origin of the word "mouse," which originated from the Sanskrit "mush," meaning "to steal".[9] Mice were known to raid grain larders and to spread disease, leading to their status as vermin throughout the Western world. Mice were viewed more favorably, however, in portions of Asia, where the observation of variants differing in appearance and behavior led to the domestication of unusual mice as pets. Records from 80 B.C. document the existence of mice bred by Japanese mouse enthusiasts who were entertained by their displays of hyperactivity, circling, and head tossing (the behavior of these animals, the likely consequence of inner ear degeneration, led to their later popularization and designation as "waltzing mice").[9, 10] In the early 19th century, traders transported unusual "fancy" mice from Asia to Europe, where mouse "fanciers" developed many unique varieties by crossing European and Asian subspecies. The popularity of fancy mice in England was illustrated by the establishment of a London "National Mouse Club" that set standards for "show mice" and held contests, awarding prizes for varieties such as white sables, satins, creamy buffs, and ruby-eyed yellows and an overall prize for "best in show."[9, 11, 12]

With the rediscovery of Mendel's laws in 1900, Harvard biologist

William Ernest Castle became interested in the extent to which coat color inheritance in fancy mice resembled the patterns of pea color heritability described by Mendel. Castle obtained animals from the region's foremost supplier of fancy mice, retired schoolteacher Miss Abbie Lathrop of Granby, Mass., whose mouse farm contained more than 11,000 mice (priced at $10–$20 per hundred).[13] Castle's initial studies of the "experimental evolution" (this preceded the coining of the term "genetics" in 1908) of coat color and his role in training students in this new field earned him recognition as "the father of mammalian genetics." His students went on to rapidly characterize anomalous phenotypes other than coat color, such as short ears, shaking, hyperglycemia, dwarfism, blindness, and tumor susceptibility.[9, 13] Within several years, mice were used by Dr. Ivan Pavlov, who explored genetic influences on behavior by exposing mice to his "dinner bell" in studies of appetitive conditioning.[14]

The value of mice for genetic studies has been markedly enhanced by inbreeding strategies for the reduction of genetic heterogeneity. Mice of a particular inbred strain are essentially identical genetically, and they are homozygous (i.e., possessing two identical alleles, one on each homologous chromosome) at every genetic locus. The availability of genetically homogeneous populations of mice is highly beneficial for minimizing the extent to which genetic factors contribute to variability in responses to experimental manipulations. Moreover, each inbred strain possesses a unique, fixed set of alleles resulting in distinct biological properties (also known as "phenotypes"), such as variations in coat color, size, cancer susceptibility, and behavioral traits. Phenotypic differences between inbred strains may be examined in an effort to identify the genetic differences that underlie them. Since the generation of the first inbred mouse strain in 1909, over 450 inbred strains have been developed, contributing to advances throughout biomedical research and to work that has resulted in at least 17 Nobel prizes.[11, 15] To this day, most of the strains in common use have ancestors from Abbie Lathrop's mouse farm.[13]

In addition to the reasons just described, practical considerations have also contributed to the popularity of laboratory mice for mammalian genetic studies. Like many small rodent species, they are proficient breeders—their gestation period is 3 weeks, and they are reproductively competent by 6–7 weeks of age. In practice, a breeding program can produce five generations of mice per year, while their small size allows for the economical maintenance of large numbers of animals in group-housing conditions. The development of procedures rendering the mouse genome accessible to experimental manipulation has catalyzed a recent rapid acceleration in the use of mice. Current methods permit the generation of mice bearing mutations of virtually any gene. The elucidation of the mouse genome, coupled with the availability of new molecular technologies enabling examination of genetic influences on behavior, provides unique opportunities to advance psychiatric research. The wide variety of mouse molecular genetic approaches and their application to the study of neural processes relevant to psychiatric illnesses will be discussed.

Relevance of Mouse Behavior to Psychiatric Phenomenology: Our "Inner Mice"

The adult mouse brain is approximately the size of a garbanzo bean—possessing a mass less than 1/2000 that of the human brain. The brains and behavioral patterns of the two species have diverged substantially, in accord with their distinctive ecological niches. The elaboration of the human cerebral cortex and other evolutionary adaptations have contributed to the considerable complexity of human cognitive capacities, affective regulation, social interactions, and societal structures. The relatively modest cortices and communication skills of mice restrict their use as plausible models for psychological processes such as artistic creativity, grief, body image, or dynamic psychotherapy. In light of these obvious species differences, what evidence exists that an understanding of mouse brain function may be pertinent to human behavior and psychiatric disease?

The human cerebral cortex does not function in isolation—it is intimately interconnected with subcortical structures that are well conserved across mammalian species. The brains of vertebrates have a common structural organization, consisting of the cerebral hemispheres, diencephalon, midbrain, cerebellum, pons, and medulla.[16] Among mammals, and frequently across other vertebrate classes, the neural structures within these divisions and the circuits that interconnect them have extensive similarities. For example, the substantia nigra appears in reptilian evolution, and this nucleus has a similar organization among marsupial and placental mammals, including a pars compacta subdivision containing dopaminergic neurons displaying similar patterns of projections to terminal fields.[16]

Despite the differing lifestyles of humans and mice, their extensive genetic and neuroanatomical homologies give rise to a wide variety of behavioral processes that are well conserved between species. Exploration of these shared brain functions—our "inner mice"—will shed light on fundamental elements of human behavioral regulation. For example, both humans and mice display complex processes such as hunger, fear, aggression, sleep, circadian rhythms, classical and operant conditioning, and sexual behavior. Functional homologies between species frequently generalize to behavioral responses to drugs—sedative, activating, anorectic, rewarding—and other behavioral properties of drugs observed in humans are frequently found in mice. Such species similarities in behavioral pharmacology are recognized by the pharmaceutical industry, for which rodent behavioral assays are an important component of the psychiatric drug discovery process.

Just as behavioral responses to drugs may generalize across species, so may behavioral responses to genetic perturbations. For example, an X-linked pattern of inheritance was noted in males of a Dutch family for a behavioral disturbance characterized by impulsive aggressiveness and impulsive sexual approaches to females. The syndrome was subsequently attributed to a point mutation in the gene encoding monoamine oxidase A (MAOA) that markedly reduced its function.[17] Quite by chance, a similar behavioral syndrome was unintentionally engineered in mice. A line of mice bearing a gene encoding interferon was generated for immunological studies, but investigators observed a phenotype difficult to ascribe to interferon function. When males were group-housed, mutants displayed elevated aggression, resulting in a large number of wounded animals.[18] Moreover, the mutant males displayed frequent attempts to grasp and mate with unreceptive females. Further analysis revealed that the interferon transgene had randomly integrated into and disrupted the MAOA gene, leading to a behavioral syndrome mimicking that seen in the Dutch family.

The potential for mouse models to reproduce aspects of complex neuropsychiatric disorders is further illustrated by studies of mutant mice lacking the hypothalamic neuropeptide orexin.[19] These animals displayed a dramatic behavioral syndrome, characterized by frequent episodes of inactivity that were manifested by the sudden collapse of the head and buckling of extremities. EEG analysis revealed instances in which the attacks were accompanied by sudden transitions from wakefulness into REM sleep, a phenomenon observed in human narcolepsy and in a strain of narcoleptic Doberman pinschers. Moreover, a mutation of an orexin receptor gene was found to underlie the canine syndrome.[20] On the basis of these findings, the orexin system was examined in narcoleptic patients, and profound orexin deficiencies were observed.[21, 22] Thus, studies of orexin-deficient mutant mice revealed a novel role for orexin in the regulation of arousal and an important animal model for examining the pathophysiology and treatment of a neuropsychiatric disorder with complex behavioral manifestations.

These examples illustrate that, in some instances, perturbations of neural genes will produce similar behavioral outcomes in mice and humans. In other cases, however, the consequences of neural mutations will bear little resemblance between species. For example, disparities in behavioral response flexibility attributable to species differences in cortical and other neural specializations could enable humans but not mice to compensate for some mutations of neural genes. Conversely, the neurobehavioral consequences of some mutations may be more readily detected in humans, because of the availability of self-report data and stringent functional requirements imposed on the human nervous system by societal demands. It is notable that species differences in the phenotypic consequences of mutations are not unique to behavior, as evidenced by the marked differences in the lung pathology produced by cystic fibrosis gene mutations across species.[23] Despite these discrepancies, mutant mice remain valuable for examining the normal function of this gene and for exploring the genetic interactions and species differences that influence the severity of pulmonary phenotypes. Similarly, examination of factors accounting for species differences in behavioral responses to mutations would provide valuable lines of research.

Modifying the Mouse Genome

The diverse strategies used to modify the mouse genome may be considered to fall within two broad categories. The first includes approaches for introducing known genetic mutations and examining their phenotypic consequences in the resulting animals. Most commonly, transgenic and gene targeting approaches are used to generate lines of mice with enhanced, reduced, or altered gene expression. The second category consists of "phenotype-based" approaches, used for identifying genes that contribute to phenotypic differences observed between inbred strains and to phenotypic abnormalities resulting from the induction of random mutations.

Mice Bearing Mutations of Known Genes

Transgenic Technology

Two decades ago, procedures were developed for introducing engineered DNA ("transgenes") into the mouse genome for the generation of transgenic mice. Thousands of lines of transgenic mice have been generated with this procedure, which has become the most commonly used technique for genetic manipulation in the mouse. Transgenic

DNA constructs commonly consist of a gene of interest linked to "promoter" sequences that direct the anatomical distribution and timing of transgene expression. These constructs are introduced by microinjection into fertilized mouse eggs, which are then surgically transferred to foster mothers. Often, transgenes integrate at a single random chromosomal location in multiple copies, permitting high levels of transgene expression. The resulting transgenic mice may be used as "founders," which are then bred to transmit the transgene to the next generation. In a small proportion of cases, phenotypes of transgenic mice may result from a transgene inserting into and disrupting the function of a native gene (as was the case for the MAOA mutant described earlier). Controls must therefore be performed to determine the extent to which a phenotype is attributable to the transgene, rather than to its genomic site of integration.

Transgenic techniques may be employed in a wide variety of experimental strategies. Because transgenic mice often possess multiple copies of the transgene, they may be used to examine the consequences of enhancing the function of a particular gene of interest through its "overexpression." It is also possible to reduce gene function by engineering "dominant negative" mutations that encode proteins designed to interfere with the function of the native gene product. Transgenic procedures may also be used to investigate the roles of particular neuronal cell types by selectively directing expression of genes that alter their function. For example, a transgenic line was developed in which the promoter for the D_1 dopamine receptor was used to drive expression of an activating protein to stimulate cells that express D_1 dopamine receptors. Chronic overstimulation of forebrain neurons expressing D_1 receptors was found to produce an abnormal behavioral phenotype characterized by repetitive grooming and perseverative engagement in other motor patterns that were likened to human compulsive behaviors.[24]

Conversely, it is also possible to make cell-type–selective lesions by using DNA constructs in which cell-type–specific promoter sequences are fused to genes encoding toxic proteins. An example of this approach is represented by another line of narcoleptic mice generated to more accurately model human narcolepsy. It has been proposed that the human condition is not typically caused by mutations of orexin or its receptors but is more likely caused by an autoimmune process, resulting in the loss of hypothalamic orexin-containing neurons.[25, 26] Thus, the pathophysiology of narcolepsy may involve not only the loss of orexin but also the loss of non-orexin signaling functions of these cells. To examine the consequences of the loss of this population of neurons, a transgenic line of mice was generated in which the human orexin promoter was linked to ataxin-3, a protein that causes cell death. Thus, cells that would normally express orexin were lost in these mutants, resulting in a narcoleptic phenotype that was proposed to more accurately reflect the human condition.[27]

Additional strategies are being developed to address a caveat that is frequently pertinent to the interpretation of transgenic studies: because transgenes are commonly expressed throughout development, the resulting phenotypes could reflect either the adult function of the gene or an indirect consequence of perturbed brain development. To minimize developmental effects, "inducible" gene expression strategies have been developed that permit transgene expression to be activated or suppressed in the adult animal, at times chosen by the experimenter. For example, a line of transgenic mice has been developed with inducible expression of ΔFosB, a transcription factor implicated in behavioral responses to psychostimulants such as cocaine.[28] The expression system was designed so that chronic treatment with a tetracycline analog suppressed expression of the transgene. Following cessation of treatment in adult animals, expression levels of ΔFosB rose and were associated with increased behavioral responsiveness to cocaine. Thus, perturbations of development could be excluded as a cause of the cocaine phenotype, strengthening the contention that ΔFosB contributes to the reinforcing properties of cocaine in the normal adult brain. Descriptions of the various strategies used to achieve inducible gene expression may be found in a number of reviews.[29–31]

Gene Targeting

Another major technical advance, made in the late 1980s, was the development of gene targeting procedures enabling the precise introduction of planned mutations into predetermined sites in the mouse genome. Most frequently, mutations have been designed to generate "knockout" or "null mutant" mice, animals in which the function of an endogenous gene has been completely and selectively eliminated. Gene targeting procedures begin with the introduction of mutation-bearing DNA sequences (targeting constructs) into embryonic stem cells through exposure to an electric field.[32] Targeting constructs most commonly consist of a target gene sequence into which a loss-of-function ("null") mutation has been engineered. They are designed to precisely replace the homologous (matching) native gene sequence within the genome. Embryonic stem cell clones in which this replacement event has occurred are identified and used to generate mice. They are microinjected into the fluid-filled cavity of 3–4-day-old mouse embryos, which are then surgically transferred to surrogate mothers that give birth to "chimeric" mice that are partly derived from the injected embryonic stem cells and partly derived from the host embryos. Chimeras are bred with animals lacking the mutation, and genomic DNA obtained from the progeny is screened for germ line transmission of the mutation. The resulting mice are bred to produce homozygous mutant (bearing two copies of the mutant gene), knockout mice.

Since the initial knockout mice were generated, there has been exponential growth in the number of reported targeted mouse mutants.[33] Generation of knockout mice has become part of standard operating procedures for exploring the functions of genes in mammals. In cases where pharmacological agents that selectively interact with particular gene products are unavailable, examination of knockout mouse phenotypes may be the best method for uncovering their functional significance. Although a number of caveats must be considered in the interpretation of knockout phenotypes (to be discussed), they have frequently provided important insights into gene function and have predicted the actions of drugs.[34] To date, null mutations of several thousand genes have been reported, encompassing an estimated 10%–15% of the predicted gene content of the mouse genome and producing a staggering array of phenotypes involving all organ systems.[4, 33] Many lines of inbred and knockout mice are maintained by the Jackson Laboratory in Bar Harbor, Me., the world's foremost repository of genetically defined mice. They supply more than 2,500 varieties to the research community and currently list 484 strains with phenotypes relevant to the study of nervous system function.

The potential of knockout mice to shed light on gene functions relevant to behavioral disorders is illustrated by a line of mice lacking the 5-HT_{2C} receptor, a prominent central nervous system serotonin receptor subtype. These animals display a variety of behavioral perturbations, including an eating disorder characterized by chronic elevations of food intake, leading to late-onset ("middle-age") obesity, enhanced susceptibility to type 2 diabetes mellitus, and reduced sensitivity to the anorectic effects of the serotonergic drug dexfenfluramine.[35–38] These findings highlighted a role for 5-HT_{2C} receptors in the anorectic effects of serotonin and stimulated efforts to develop 5-HT_{2C} receptor agonists for the treatment of obesity. Further studies revealed that animals lacking this receptor displayed enhanced behavioral and neurochemical responses to cocaine, raising the possibility that 5-HT_{2C} receptor agonists might suppress the intake of psychostimulant drugs, as well as food.

Although most lines of mice generated by gene targeting have been knockouts, alternative strategies employing gene targeting are on the rise. In addition to null mutations, it is possible to introduce more subtle changes, such as point mutations that alter, but do not eliminate, gene function. For example, a single amino acid change was engineered in a gene encoding the α_1 subunit of the γ-aminobutyric acid type A (GABA$_A$) receptor, rendering GABA$_A$ receptors containing this subunit insensitive to benzodiazepines.[39-41] Whereas the resulting animals displayed reduced sensitivity to the sedative and amnestic effects of diazepam, no change in sensitivity to the anxiolytic-like effects of this drug was observed. By contrast, mice bearing a corresponding mutation in the α_2 subunit were insensitive to the anxiolytic-like effects of diazepam. These results indicate a strategy for anxiolytic drug development. Benzodiazepine site ligands active at α_2-containing GABA$_A$ receptors, while devoid of activity at receptors containing the α_1 subunit, may produce anxiolytic effects without some of the side effects typically associated with benzodiazepines.[41]

Additional advances in gene targeting technologies will allow for cell-type–specific and temporal control of gene expression. In standard knockout mouse lines, the normal gene product is completely absent throughout development from all of the regions in which it is normally expressed. It may therefore be difficult to precisely identify the critical neural circuits through which a mutation alters behavior and the developmental time period in which the mutation produces its effect. To address this problem, "conditional" gene targeting approaches have been devised for the restriction of targeted mutations to subpopulations of cells or for the induction of mutations at predetermined developmental stages. Descriptions of procedures for conditional gene targeting are beyond the scope of this discussion, but recent reviews are available.[31, 42]

Phenotype-Based Approaches

In contrast to transgenic and gene targeting approaches, which are often used to explore the function of known genes, phenotype-based approaches work in reverse: phenotypes that exist in particular inbred strains or in animals with induced mutations are subjected to genetic analysis in an effort to identify the genes that contribute to the phenotype. Two approaches in common use are quantitative trait locus and random mutagenesis strategies.

Quantitative Trait Locus Analysis

A quantitative trait locus is a chromosomal region containing a gene (or genes) that contributes a portion of the genetic variation of a quantifiable phenotype. Commonly, mouse quantitative trait locus studies are undertaken to identify "naturally occurring" genetic variations that underlie known phenotypic differences between two inbred strains of mice. For example, one strain of mice may score high and another strain low on a behavioral measure associated with anxiety. Typically, the two strains are interbred, creating a generation of hybrid mice designated F1. The F1 animals are then crossed to produce an F2 generation composed of mice with varying contributions of genes from the two parental strains, due to genetic recombination during gamete formation.

In this example, the F2 mice would then be tested in the anxiety assay that distinguished the two parental strains. A continuous distribution of behavioral scores is usually found, and animals at the extremes of the distribution are selected for further genetic analysis. Correlations are sought between the behavioral scores and the inheritance patterns of genetic markers that are "polymorphic," i.e., that differ between strains. DNA polymorphisms termed "simple sequence length polymorphisms," or "SSLPs," are widely distributed throughout the genome, are readily detected, and may thus serve as markers. Quantitative trait locus analyses are performed by using a variety of statistical techniques to test the probability that variation in the phenotype is associated with a particular mapped marker. Following identification of quantitative trait loci that contribute significantly to phenotypic variation, a variety of strategies are employed to precisely identify the gene bearing the functional variant. Approaches include analysis of previously unknown genes in the quantitative trait locus region, sequencing of known candidate genes, and determination of differential gene expression. Detailed descriptions of theory and practice are available.[43, 44]

Quantitative trait locus analyses allow for the identification of genes influencing phenotypic variation without a priori knowledge of the genes themselves. This is particularly advantageous for the study of complex behaviors, since the genes most relevant to phenotypic variation in neural processes regulating behavior remain unclear. Several limitations to this approach also warrant consideration. For traits that are regulated by a very large number of genes with small effects, very large sample sizes may be required. In addition, quantitative trait locus analysis cannot be used to screen for all genes that are essential to neurobiological pathways regulating behavior. It is restricted to alleles that happen to differ between the two parental strains. Quantitative trait locus analyses have been performed with limited success to identify genes contributing to a large number of neurobehavioral processes, such as anxiety regulation, learning, seizure sensitivity, sensorimotor gating, and responses to drugs of abuse.[32]

Random Mutagenesis

An alternative phenotype-based genomic screening approach has recently attracted much attention and investment. Efforts are underway to generate large numbers of animals bearing random single-base-pair mutations for screening in a wide variety of phenotypic assays. Mutations are induced chemically, by treating male mice with N-ethyl-N-nitrosourea to induce single-base-pair mutations in the spermatogonia.[45] These mice are then bred, and offspring are screened for phenotypes of interest. Because all mutations in this generation of mice would be in the heterozygous state, phenotypic screening would detect only dominant mutations. To detect recessive mutations (mutations that produce phenotypic abnormalities only in the homozygous state), additional crosses would be required to generate and screen offspring that are homozygous for induced mutations, an expensive task. The doses of N-ethyl-N-nitrosourea typically employed result in animals with multiple mutations—it has been estimated that 650 lines of the resulting mice are sufficient to obtain animals with null mutations of 15,000 genes (50% coverage of the genome).

The screening of mutagenized mice typically involves assessment in a battery of physiological and behavioral assays. When testing for behavioral phenotypes, it is important to recognize that the induced mutations are random and not restricted to genes regulating the behavioral process of interest.[45] For example, genetic perturbations producing illness, motor impairment, cognitive perturbations, blindness, or olfaction deficits could alter behavior in an assay intended to assess anxiety. Therefore, tests of peripheral organ system function and a global neurological assessment are usually incorporated in the primary mutagenesis screen. Although many mice are generated by the mutagenesis procedure, practical considerations allow testing of only a small number of mice bearing each unique complement of mutations, limiting statistical power in detecting phenotypic alterations. Therefore, investigators tend to focus on mice with scores near the extremes of the population distribution for the phenotypic assay of interest. Progeny of mice bearing true positive mutations will transmit the altered trait between generations. Once identified, the mutations are localized to chromosomal regions by using gene mapping methods. Ultimately, the actual mutation is identified through demonstration of a sequence difference that tracks with the phenotype.

The potential utility of the random mutagenesis approach has been demonstrated by studies of mice bearing mutations of the *Clock* gene. In a search for genes influencing circadian rhythms, investigators used

N-ethyl-N-nitrosourea mutagenesis and screened animals for genetic influences on wheel-running, a diurnally regulated behavior used to assess circadian rhythmicity. A mutation was found that in the heterozygous state lengthened the circadian period of wheel-running behavior and in the homozygous state led to the loss of circadian rhythmicity altogether.[47] The responsible mutation was mapped, and the *Clock* gene was molecularly cloned.[48] Further characterization revealed the gene to be expressed in the suprachiasmatic nucleus, a hypothalamic region implicated in circadian rhythm regulation. This work set the stage for studies that are providing novel insights into neural mechanisms that underlie circadian rhythms. Subsequent enthusiasm for chemical mutagenesis approaches has led to the establishment of several international centers devoted to mutagenesis screens.[4, 49] It is anticipated that current large-scale efforts will result in thousands of single-gene mutants, many of which will provide novel insights into neural processes that regulate behavior. In addition to chemical methods for inducing mutations, alternative approaches, such as "gene trapping," are being developed to facilitate identification and characterization of randomly induced mutations.[50]

Evaluating Mouse Behavioral Models of Psychiatric Illnesses

The rigorous design and implementation of procedures for analyzing mouse behavior are critical for translating the rapid advances in mammalian genomics into insights relevant to psychiatric disease pathophysiology and treatment. Confusion regarding the interpretation of mouse behavioral tests may be reduced by carefully considering the varying purposes for which particular assays are used. Willner[51] has proposed categorization of behavioral assays into three classes: 1) behavioral bioassays, 2) screening tests, and 3) models (simulations) of clinical conditions. Behavioral bioassays utilize behavior as an output measure to assess particular physiological processes. For example, the influence of drugs on the nigrostriatal dopamine system has been assessed by examining their effects on circling behavior in animals that had received unilateral dopamine system lesions. In an analogous fashion, head-twitch responses have been used as a measure of the ability of compounds to act as serotonin receptor agonists. The results of such behavioral bioassays are interpreted with regard to discrete physiological processes rather than to clinical conditions.

Behavioral screening tests are commonly used in the pharmaceutical industry for their "predictive validity"—i.e., the likelihood that the effects of compounds in the assay will predict their efficacy for the treatment of particular psychiatric disorders. A test may be useful for this purpose regardless of whether it appears to accurately reproduce the cause or symptoms of the disorder. For example, the two most frequently used depression-related mouse behavioral tests are the forced swim and the tail suspension "behavioral despair" assays. The forced swim test is conducted by placing animals for several minutes in a water-containing cylinder from which they cannot escape. Initially, mice display high levels of activity in apparent escape attempts, which decrease in frequency as the animals exhibit episodes of immobility during which they appear to float at the surface. This immobile state was initially proposed to reflect "behavioral despair"—the loss of hope of escaping.[52] Because immobility in this assay is reduced by a wide variety of antidepressant drugs, the assay is used in the pharmaceutical industry to predict potential antidepressant efficacy of novel compounds. A variant of this assay, the tail suspension test, is more sensitive to serotonergic antidepressants.[53] In this test, animals are suspended by the tail for several minutes, and the time spent immobile (without apparent escape attempts) is measured. Mutations of a number of genes implicated in antidepressant action have been associated with abnormal responses in these tests, including those encoding the serotonin 5-HT_{1A} and 5-HT_{1B} receptors, α-adrenergic receptors, monoamine oxidases A and B, and the norepinephrine plasma membrane transporter.[53]

Can one conclude that a mouse displaying elevated immobility in these tests is "depressed"? Mice are notoriously noncompliant with questionnaires and interviews, precluding collection of the kinds of self-report data upon which much of psychiatric diagnosis is based. Perturbations of psychological processes must be inferred from behavior, and consideration of the validity of behavioral assays is essential to their interpretation. The "face validity" of the forced swim test, i.e., the degree to which a floating mouse resembles a depressed individual, is limited. It could also be argued that its "construct validity," i.e., the extent to which the assay reproduces the etiology and pathophysiology of depression, is also questionable. It is unclear that immobility in this assay reflects a state of "despair," because immobility may be alternatively viewed as a reasonably adaptive strategy for coping with this experimental situation. In view of these caveats, a conservative interpretation of an elevated immobility result would be warranted. Rather than surmising that the mouse is depressed, it would be more appropriate to conclude that the mouse has an abnormality of a behavior associated with responsiveness to antidepressants. Despite these considerations, the significant predictive validity of the forced swim and tail suspension tests indicates that insights into the mechanisms under-lying such a behavioral phenotype may shed light on the function of neural pathways pertinent to the treatment of depression.

Another class of behavioral assays with substantial predictive valid-ity are used to model anxiety states.[54] The most frequently employed class of tests assesses exploratory behavior, relying on the innate predis-position of rodents to avoid open and/or brightly lit spaces—presum-ably an innate response evolved to minimize the risk of predation. For example, when placed in a novel behavioral enclosure, mice exhibit an affinity for the periphery of the behavioral arena rather than the center. The proportion of time spent in the periphery is proposed to correlate with anxiety state. The most commonly used screening test for examin-ing the effects of experimental manipulations on anxiety-like behavior is the elevated "plus" maze. This consists of an elevated platform that is shaped like a plus symbol, with four arms, two of which are walled and two open. The predisposition of mice to prefer the closed to the open arms is proposed to correlate with anxiety state. The effects of pharmacological agents in this assay are predictive of their anxiolytic efficacy in humans. Thus, diazepam increases the proportion of time animals spend exploring the open arms. Conversely, *m*-chlorophenyl-piperazine, a nonselective serotonin receptor agonist, reduces explora-tion of the open arms and produces anxiogenic responses in humans.

To date, behavioral abnormalities consistent with the dysregulation of anxiety have been reported in at least 30 lines of mice.[55] For example, marked enhancements of anxiety-related behaviors were observed in three different laboratories that independently generated mice bearing a targeted null mutation of the serotonin 5-HT_{1A} receptor gene.[56-58] This phenotype is consistent with the known anxiolytic properties of 5-HT_{1A} receptor partial agonists, such as buspirone. These mutants may be used to examine mechanisms through which serotonin systems regu-late anxiety. Behavioral analysis of animals bearing mutations affecting the signaling of corticotropin-releasing factor (CRF) also reveals results consistent with its proposed role in anxiety regulation. Thus, elevated anxiety-like behaviors were observed in mice bearing mutations en-hancing CRF expression,[59] and reductions of such behaviors were ex-hibited in mice with genetic perturbations reducing brain CRF signaling.[60] Mutations impacting the signaling of acetylcholine, dopa-mine, GABA, neuropeptide Y, cholecystokinin, nitric oxide, and other neuromodulators have also been found to impact anxiety-related be-haviors.[55]

It is noteworthy that the assays of rodent depression- and anxiety-related behavior just discussed may be considered to model particular behavioral states rather than the full range of affective, cognitive, and neurovegetative symptoms characteristic of common psychiatric disorders. As discussed in other contributions to this issue, susceptibilities to these illnesses are polygenically determined, and the environmental contributions to their pathophysiology are incompletely understood. Therefore, current mouse models may be most productively used to examine the biological bases of individual features of psychiatric disorders rather than as comprehensive models of complex psychiatric syndromes.[54] Exceptions to this are conditions in which clear etiological factors have been identified. In the case of substance use disorders, an important etiological factor, the abused drug, is known. Thus, studies may be performed in which a wide variety of physiological and behavioral responses to the abused substance are examined. In addition, as genetic factors conferring susceptibility to psychiatric diseases are uncovered, it will be possible to perform detailed analyses of the phenotypic consequences of their introduction into the mouse genome.

Priorities for the Development of Neurobehavioral Assessment Strategies in the Mouse

Procedures for the manipulation of the mouse genome are continuing to develop at a rapid pace and are becoming increasingly accessible to investigators. With the development of large-scale mouse mutagenesis programs and the proliferation of inbred, transgenic, knockout, and other genetically modified strains, we have become inundated with valuable mutant mice. The extent to which mouse genetic approaches will provide insights into the neural bases of psychiatric disorders rests critically on the ability to examine the influence of mutations on complex behavior. Unfortunately, technology development for mouse behavioral analysis has lagged behind the pace of innovation in mammalian genetics and genomics. Many of the behavioral assays in common use were originally designed for rats several decades ago and have been recently adapted to mice with little change other than reductions in equipment dimensions. Existing behavioral testing procedures can be time- and labor-intensive, and many factors may complicate their interpretation. These limitations have contributed to a substantial bottleneck in our ability to make maximal use of advances in mouse genome manipulation to study the neural basis of mammalian behavior. The field is currently in its infancy, and its development would be furthered by progress in a number of areas.

Standardization of Equipment and Experimental Procedures

Currently, many aspects of behavioral testing equipment and procedures are not standardized among laboratories.[61] For example, physical features of the elevated plus maze such as dimensions, color, and construction material may differ, contributing to avoidable interlaboratory variability. In addition, procedural differences in the conduct of behavioral assays may vary between laboratories. Often, overlooked variables such as mouse-handling practices, housing conditions, and testing room environments may influence results. Consensus on sets of standard procedures is required, along with enhanced appreciation of the extent to which uncontrolled environmental variables may influence behavioral performance.

Diagnostic Standards

Currently, there are no standards to which investigators can refer to draw conclusions about the behavioral traits of their mutants. As a consequence, some investigators may report a behavioral phenotype based on a single marginal assay, whereas others maintain more stringent criteria. In the absence of clear diagnostic standards, a conservative approach would be to require a consistent pattern of abnormal behavioral responses across several assays pertinent to a given behavioral domain before conclusions are drawn.

Need to Assess Multiple Behavioral Domains

Principles of clinical evaluation can be useful in the analysis of mutant mouse phenotypes. For example, clinicians do not limit their inquiries to the chief complaint, and they perform a review of systems to minimize the risk of overlooking important information. However, investigators interested in a particular behavioral trait sometimes perform a very restricted analysis, limited to the behavioral domain of interest. This could be problematic because an undetected deficit in another behavioral domain could influence the interpretation of results. For example, an animal with normal trait anxiety could perform abnormally on the elevated plus maze because of an undetected cognitive deficit. Conversely, a mouse with a motor impairment or a severe stress response to a learning task may perform abnormally for reasons other than cognitive impairment. Thus, the exploration of multiple behavioral domains will maximize the extent to which each individual assay may be correctly interpreted.

Limitations of Behavioral Batteries

To maximize the information that can be obtained from limited numbers of mutants, cohorts of mice are often examined in a battery of behavioral tests requiring repeated removal from their home cages. Implementation of behavioral batteries may be associated with drawbacks that are difficult to avoid, such as 1) they are time-consuming and labor-intensive, 2) the order of test administration can skew the resulting data, and 3) repeated removal of mice from the home cage produces stress that may confound interpretation of behavioral data. These problems may be addressed by use of experimental designs that control for test order and by the development of alternative behavioral analysis strategies permitting simultaneous assessment of multiple behaviors, as will be described.

Strain Information

The large number of available inbred strains represents a resource that has yet to be fully utilized. Although inbred strains are known to display a wide variety of behavioral phenotypes, these have not been systematically characterized. To address this issue, a large-scale international "Mouse Phenome Project" has been recently initiated by the Jackson Laboratory to establish a database containing detailed phenotypic information (behavioral and nonbehavioral) from a wide variety of inbred strains.[62] Such information may be used for the purpose of selecting strains with characteristics most suitable for investigating particular mutant phenotypes or for identifying strain differences in traits of interest for quantitative trait locus studies.

Need for Assays of Additional Behaviors

The development of satisfactory animal models that simultaneously mimic multiple features of complex psychiatric disorders of uncertain etiology may be extremely difficult. However, it may be feasible to develop new assays relevant to particular features of psychiatric illnesses that are not commonly modeled in mice, such as compulsions, panic attacks, binge eating, impulsivity, distractibility, and anhedonia. In some cases, useful assays that have been previously established in rats could be adapted to mice. In other cases, novel approaches will be required.

Gene-Environment Interactions

Susceptibility to psychiatric illnesses depends not only on genetic endowment but also on experience. Although mouse genetic studies most commonly focus on the influences of genes, they may also be used to explore the interactions between genes and environment on the establishment of behavioral traits. For example, rodent behavior is susceptible to social influences, as demonstrated by studies revealing that a mother's treatment of her pups can produce lifelong influences on stress reactivity in her offspring.[63] Mouse molecular genetic approaches may be applied to determine the influence of genes both on maternal behavior and on the sensitivity of pups to experimental perturbations of the maternal care they receive. Genetic influences on the behavioral consequences of a wide range of additional environmental factors, including chronic stress, social defeat, diet, and environmental enrichment, also warrant further exploration in the mouse.

Behavioral Assays Applied to Both Humans and Mice

A challenge in determining the relevance of animal studies to psychiatric conditions results from fundamental differences in the nature of the data used for assessment of psychological processes in humans and mice. While psychiatric assessment relies heavily on self-report data, assessment of psychological processes in mice requires inferences derived from the analysis of behavior. Although the prospects of obtaining useful self-report data from mice remain discouraging, there is increasing interest in the development of behavioral assays that may be applied to both mice and humans. One example is the prepulse inhibition assay, which examines the ability of a sensory stimulus to suppress the startle response to a subsequent stimulus. This index of sensorimotor gating is perturbed in schizophrenia, and the effects of drugs on prepulse inhibition are similar in mice and human subjects.[64] Many possibilities exist for the development of new cross-species assays that may be applied to additional domains of behavior.

Need for Technological Innovations for Behavioral Assessment

New technologies that have revolutionized genomics and other scientific fields may also be used to develop novel approaches for behavioral assessment—the application of advances in information technology may be particularly useful. Toward this end, my colleagues and I, as well as others, are combining automated behavioral data collection systems with sophisticated computational tools for "behavioral informatics" approaches to phenotype analysis. The spontaneous behavior patterns exhibited by mice in their home cages provide a rich source of information reflecting the functional output of the brain. Behaviors such as exploration, feeding, drinking, sleeping, grooming, and diurnal rhythms reflect the functions of numerous neuronal pathways, each influenced by large numbers of genes. Rather than removing animals from their home cages and isolating various behavioral domains in individual tests, this approach will entail the introduction of experimental manipulations into the home cage. Their impact may thus be examined in the context of the integrated expression of multiple behavioral domains ("mouse lifestyles"), reflecting the outputs of multiple neuronal pathways. We have been developing such technology with the goal of systematically establishing a database recording the impact of genes, drugs, environmental exposures, and brain lesions on spontaneous behavioral patterns. Such a resource will provide a sensitive tool for assessment of the neurobehavioral consequences of mutations and other experimental manipulations. We anticipate many such new technology initiatives will be developed in academic and industrial settings. Such efforts, along with progress in meeting the multiple challenges already outlined, will permit a detailed assessment of brain function in the mouse and enhance the extent to which the revolution in mouse molecular genetics will benefit psychiatric research.

References

1. Battey J, Jordan E, Cox D, Dove W: An action plan for mouse genomics. Nat Genet 1999; 21:73–75
2. Waterston RH, Lindblad-Toh K, Birney E, Rogers J, Abril JF, Agarwal P, Agarwala R, Ainscough R, Alexandersson M, An P, Antonarakis SE, Attwood J, et al: Initial sequencing and comparative analysis of the mouse genome. Nature 2002; 420:520–562
3. Boguski MS: Comparative genomics: the mouse that roared. Nature 2002; 420:515–516
4. Bradley A: Mining the mouse genome. Nature 2002; 420:512–514
5. Madsen O, Scally M, Douady CJ, Kao DJ, DeBry RW, Adkins R, Amrine HM, Stanhope MJ, de Jong WW, Springer MS: Parallel adaptive radiations in two major clades of placental mammals. Nature 2001; 409:610–614
6. Murphy WJ, Eizirik E, Johnson WE, Zhang YP, Ryder OA, O'Brien SJ: Molecular phylogenetics and the origins of placental mammals. Nature 2001; 409:614–618
7. Gunter C, Dhand R: Human biology by proxy. Nature 2002; 420:509
8. Nadeau JH: Single nucleotide polymorphisms: tackling complexity. Nature 2002; 420:517–518

9. Foster HL, Small JD, Fox JG: The Mouse in Biomedical Research. New York, Academic Press, 1981

10. Searle AG, Lyon MF, International Committee on Standardized Genetic Nomenclature for Mice: Genetic Variants and Strains of the Laboratory Mouse. New York, Oxford University Press, 1989

11. Beck JA, Lloyd S, Hafezparast M, Lennon-Pierce M, Eppig JT, Festing MF, Fisher EM: Genealogies of mouse inbred strains. Nat Genet 2000; 24:23–25

12. Wade CM, Kulbokas EJ III, Kirby AW, Zody MC, Mullikin JC, Lander ES, Lindblad-Toh K, Daly MJ: The mosaic structure of variation in the laboratory mouse genome. Nature 2002; 420:574–578

13. Morse HC III (ed): Origins of Inbred Mice. New York, Academic Press, 1978

14. Krushinsky LV, Molodkina LN, Gless DA, Dobrokhotova LP, Steshenko AP, Semiokhina AF, Zorina ZA, Romanova LG: The functional state of the brain during sonic stimulation, in Physiological Effects of Noise. Edited by Welch BL, Welch AS. New York, Plenum, 1970, pp 159–183

15. Festing MFW, Fisher EMC: Mighty mice. Nature 2000; 404:815

16. Sarnat HB, Netsky MG: Evolution of the Nervous System. New York, Oxford University Press, 1981

17. Brunner HG, Nelen M, Breakefield XO, Ropers HH, van Oost BA: Abnormal behavior associated with a point mutation in the structural gene for monoamine oxidase A. Science 1993; 262:578–580

18. Cases O, Seif I, Grimsby J, Gaspar P, Chen K, Pournin S, Müller U, Aguet M, Babinet C, Shih J, De Maeyer E: Aggressive behavior and altered amounts of brain serotonin and norepinephrine in mice lacking MAOA. Science 1995; 268:1763–1766

19. Chemelli RM, Willie JT, Sinton CM, Elmquist JK, Scammell T, Lee C, Richardson JA, Williams SC, Xiong Y, Kisanuki Y, Fitch TE, Nakazato M, Hammer RE, Saper CB, Yanagisawa M: Narcolepsy in orexin knockout mice: molecular genetics of sleep regulation. Cell 1999; 98:437–451

20. Lin L, Faraco J, Li R, Kadotani H, Rogers W, Lin X, Qiu X, de Jong PJ, Nishino S, Mignot E: The sleep disorder canine narcolepsy is caused by a mutation in the hypocretin (orexin) receptor 2 gene. Cell 1999; 98:365–376

21. Nishino S, Ripley B, Overeem S, Lammers GJ, Mignot E: Hypocretin (orexin) deficiency in human narcolepsy (letter). Lancet 2000; 355:39–40

22. Peyron C, Faraco J, Rogers W, Ripley B, Overeem S, Charnay Y, Nevsimalova S, Aldrich M, Reynolds D, Albin R, Li R, Hungs M, Pedrazzoli M, Padigaru M, Kucherlapati M, Fan J, Maki R, Lammers GJ, Bouras C, Kucherlapati R, Nishino S, Mignot E: A mutation in a case of early onset narcolepsy and a generalized absence of hypocretin peptides in human narcoleptic brains. Nat Med 2000; 6:991–997

23. Davidson DJ, Rolfe M: Mouse models of cystic fibrosis. Trends Genet 2001; 17(Oct suppl):S29–S37

24. Campbell KM, de Lecea L, Severynse DM, Caron MG, McGrath MJ, Spar- ber SB, Sun LY, Burton FH: OCD-like behaviors caused by a neuropoten- tiating transgene targeted to cortical and limbic D1+ neurons. J Neurosci 1999; 19:5044–5053

25. Peyron C, Faraco J, Rogers W, Ripley B, Overeem S, Charnay Y, Nevsi- malova S, Aldrich M, Reynolds D, Albin R, Li R, Hungs M, Pedrazzoli M, Padigaru M, Kucherlapati M, Fan J, Maki R, Lammers GJ, Bouras C, Kucherlapati R, Nishino S, Mignot E: A mutation in a case of early onset narcolepsy and a generalized absence of hypocretin peptides in human narcoleptic brains. Nat Med 2000; 6:991–997

26. Thannickal TC, Moore RY, Nienhuis R, Ramanathan L, Gulyani S, Ald- rich M, Cornford M, Siegel JM: Reduced number of hypocretin neurons in human narcolepsy. Neuron 2000; 27:469–474

27. Hara J, Beuckmann CT, Nambu T, Willie JT, Chemelli RM, Sinton CM, Sugiyama F, Yagami K, Goto K, Yanagisawa M, Sakurai T: Genetic abla- tion of orexin neurons in mice results in narcolepsy, hypophagia, and obesity. Neuron 2001; 30:345–354

28. Kelz MB, Chen J, Carlezon WA Jr, Whisler K, Gilden L, Beckmann AM, Steffen C, Zhang YJ, Marotti L, Self DW, Tkatch T, Baranauskas G, Sur- meier DJ, Neve RL, Duman RS, Piccioto M, Nestler EJ: Expression of the transcription factor deltaFosB in the brain controls sensitivity to cocaine. Nature 1999; 401:272–276

29. Ryding AD, Sharp MG, Mullins JJ: Conditional transgenic technologies. J Endocrinol 2001; 171:1–14

30. Metzger D, Chambon P: Site- and time-specific gene targeting in the mouse. Methods 2001; 24:71–80

31. Lewandoski M: Conditional control of gene expression in the mouse. Nat Rev Genet 2001; 2:743–755

32. Tecott LH, Wehner JM: Mouse molecular genetic technologies: promise for psychiatric research. Arch Gen Psychiatry 2001; 58:995–1004

33. Muller U: Ten years of gene targeting: targeted mouse mutants, from vec- tor design to phenotype analysis. Mech Dev 1999; 82:3–21

34. Zambrowicz BP, Sands AT: Knockouts model the 100 best-selling drugs—will they model the next 100? Nat Rev Drug Discov 2003; 2:38–51

35. Tecott LH, Sun LM, Akana SF, Strack AM, Lowenstein DH, Dallman MF, Julius D: Eating disorder and epilepsy in mice lacking 5HT2C serotonin receptors. Nature 1995; 374:542–546

36. Nonogaki K, Strack A, Dallman M, Tecott LH: Leptin-insensitive hyper- phagia and type 2 diabetes in mice with a mutated serotonin 5-HT2C re- ceptor gene. Nat Med 1998; 4:1152–1156

37. Vickers SP, Clifton PG, Dourish CT, Tecott LH: Reduced satiating effect of d-fenfluramine in serotonin 5-HT2C receptor mutant mice. Psycho- pharmacology (Berl) 1999; 143:309–314

38. Nonogaki K, Abdallah L, Goulding EH, Bonasera SJ, Tecott LH: Hyperactivity and reduced energy cost of physical activity in serotonin 5-HT(2C) receptor mutant mice. Diabetes 2003; 52:315–320

39. Rudolph U, Crestani F, Benke D, Brünig I, Benson JA, Fritschy JM, Martin JR, Bluethmann H, Möhler H: Benzodiazepine actions mediated by specific gamma-aminobutyric acid(A) receptor subtypes. Nature 1999; 401:796–800

40. McKernan RM, Rosahl TW, Reynolds DS, Sur C, Wafford KA, Atack JR, Farrar S, Myers J, Cook G, Ferris P, Garrett L, Bristow L, Marshall G, Macaulay A, Brown N, Howell O, Moore KW, Carling RW, Street LJ, Castro JL, Ragan CI, Dawson GR, Whiting PJ: Sedative but not anxiolytic properties of benzodiazepines are mediated by the GABA(A) receptor alpha1 subtype. Nat Neurosci 2000; 3:587–592

41. Rudolph U, Crestani F, Mohler H: GABA(A) receptor subtypes: dissecting their pharmacological functions. Trends Pharmacol Sci 2001; 22:188–194

42. Wells T, Carter DA: Genetic engineering of neural function in transgenic rodents: towards a comprehensive strategy? J Neurosci Methods 2001; 108:111–130

43. Belknap JK, Hitzemann R, Crabbe JC, Phillips TJ, Buck KJ, Williams RW: QTL analysis and genomewide mutagenesis in mice: complementary genetic approaches to the dissection of complex traits. Behav Genet 2001; 31:5–15

44. Crabbe JC: Genetic contributions to addiction. Annu Rev Psychol 2002; 53:435–462

45. Justice MJ, Noveroske JK, Weber JS, Zheng B, Bradley A: Mouse ENU mutagenesis. Hum Mol Genet 1999; 8:1955–1963

46. Tarantino LM, Bucan M: Dissection of behavior and psychiatric disorders using the mouse as a model. Hum Mol Genet 2000; 9:953–965

47. Vitaterna MH, King DP, Chang A-M, Kornhauser JM, Lowrey PL, McDonald JD, Dove WF, Pinto LH, Turek FW, Takahashi JS: Mutagenesis and mapping of a mouse gene, Clock, essential for circadian behavior. Science 1994; 264:719–725

48. King DP, Zhao Y, Sangoram AM, Wilsbacher LD, Tanaka M, Antoch MP, Steeves TD, Vitaterna MH, Kornhauser JM, Lowrey PL, Turek FW, Takahashi JS: Positional cloning of the mouse circadian clock gene. Cell 1997; 89:641–653

49. Nolan PM, Peters J, Strivens M, Rogers D, Hagan J, Spurr N, Gray IC, Vizor L, Brooker D, Whitehill E, Washbourne R, Hough T, Greenaway S, Hewitt M, Liu X, McCormack S, Pickford K, Selley R, Wells C, Tymowska-Lalanne Z, Roby P, Glenister P, Thornton C, Thaung C, Stevenson JA, Arkell R, Mburu P, Hardisty R, Kiernan A, Erven A, Steel KP, Voegeling S, Guenet JL, Nickols C, Sadri R, Nasse M, Isaacs A, Davies K, Browne M, Fisher EM, Martin J, Rastan S, Brown SD, Hunter J: A systematic, genome-wide, phenotype-driven mutagenesis programme for gene function studies in the mouse. Nat Genet 2000; 25:440–443

50. Munroe RJ, Bergstrom RA, Zheng QY, Libby B, Smith R, John SW, Schimenti KJ, Browning VL, Schimenti JC: Mouse mutants from chemically mutagenized embryonic stem cells. Nat Genet 2000; 24:318–321

51. Willner P: Behavioral models in psychopharmacology, in Behavioral Models in Psychopharmacology: Theoretical, Industrial and Clinical Perspectives. Edited by Willner P. Cambridge, UK, Cambridge University Press, 1991, pp 3–18

52. Porsolt RD, Le Pichon M, Jalfre M: Depression: a new animal model sensitive to antidepressant treatments. Nature 1977; 266:730–732

53. Cryan JF, Markou A, Lucki I: Assessing antidepressant activity in rodents: recent developments and future needs. Trends Pharmacol Sci 2002; 23:238–245

54. Shekhar A, McCann UD, Meaney MJ, Blanchard DC, Davis M, Frey KA, Liberzon I, Overall KL, Shear MK, Tecott LH, Winsky L: Summary of a National Institute of Mental Health workshop: developing animal models of anxiety disorders. Psychopharmacology (Berl) 2001; 157:327–339

55. Holmes A: Targeted gene mutation approaches to the study of anxiety-like behavior in mice. Neurosci Biobehav Rev 2001; 25:261–273

56. Parks CL, Robinson PS, Sibille E, Shenk T, Toth M: Increased anxiety of mice lacking the serotonin1A receptor. Proc Natl Acad Sci USA 1998; 95:10734–10739

57. Ramboz S, Oosting R, Amara DA, Kung HF, Blier P, Mendelsohn M, Mann JJ, Brunner D, Hen R: Serotonin receptor 1A knockout: an animal model of anxiety-related disorder. Proc Natl Acad Sci USA 1998; 95:14476–14481

58. Heisler L, Chu HM, Brennan T, Danao J, Bajwa P, Parsons L, Tecott LH: Elevated anxiety and antidepressant-like responses in serotonin 5-HT1A receptor mutant mice. Proc Natl Acad Sci USA 1998; 95:15049–15054

59. Stenzel-Poore MP, Heinrichs SC, Rivest S, Koob GF, Vale WW: Overproduction of corticotropin-releasing factor in transgenic mice: a genetic model of anxiogenic behavior. J Neurosci 1994; 14(5, part 1):2579–2584

60. Smith GW, Aubry JM, Dellu F, Contarino A, Bilezikjian LM, Gold LH, Chen R, Marchuk Y, Hauser C, Bentley CA, Sawchenko PE, Koob GF, Vale W, Lee KF: Corticotropin releasing factor receptor 1-deficient mice display decreased anxiety, impaired stress response, and aberrant neuroendocrine development. Neuron 1998; 20:1093–1102

61. Crabbe JC, Wahlsten D, Dudek BC: Genetics of mouse behavior: interactions with laboratory environment. Science 1999; 284:1670–1672

62. Paigen K, Eppig JT: A mouse phenome project. Mamm Genome 2000; 11:715–717

63. Meaney MJ: Maternal care, gene expression, and the transmission of individual differences in stress reactivity across generations. Annu Rev Neurosci 2001; 24:1161–1192

64. Geyer MA, Markou A: Animal models of psychiatric disorders, in Psychopharmacology: The Fourth Generation of Progress. Edited by Kupfer DJ, Bloom FE. New York, Raven Press, 1995, pp 787–798

7 Microarray Technology

A Review of New Strategies to Discover Candidate Vulnerability Genes in Psychiatric Disorders

William E. Bunney, M.D.
Blynn G. Bunney, Ph.D.
Marquis P. Vawter, Ph.D.
Hiroaki Tomita, Ph.D.
Jun Li, Ph.D.
Simon J. Evans, Ph.D.
Prabhakara V. Choudary, Ph.D.
Richard M. Myers, Ph.D.
Edward G. Jones, M.D., Ph.D.
Stanley J. Watson, M.D., Ph.D.
Huda Akil, Ph.D.

There is currently no fundamental understanding of the genes that increase the risk for psychiatric disorders. Despite success in developing new compounds based on receptor subtypes,[1, 2] a significant number of patients with these disorders remain resistant to

The authors' laboratories are supported by NIMH grants MH-54844, NS-21377, and NS-30109 (the latter two from the National Institute of Neurological and Communicative Disorders and Stroke), the W.M. Keck Foundation (to Dr. Jones), Silvio O. Conte Center grant MH-60398 (to Dr. W.E. Bunney), the Pritzker Family Philanthropic Fund, the William Lion Penzner Foundation (Dr. W.E. Bunney), and Program Project 5 MH-42251 (to Drs. Watson and Dr. Akil).

treatment,[3, 4] and there is no systematic way to determine which of a variety of treatments will be efficacious for a given patient. Limited progress has been made in identifying new and unique drug targets in these illnesses, and no objective validated diagnostic markers for these diseases have been found.[5–7]

It is now clear that psychiatric disorders such as schizophrenia and depression are not caused by a single gene abnormality but, instead, by a set of abnormal genes.[1] Complex trait disorders, such as schizophrenia and depression, are multifactorial diseases attributed to polygenic (more than a single gene) and epigenetic (e.g., changes in gene expression that are heritable but do not entail a change in DNA sequence) factors. Of the many challenges in research into complex trait disorders, one of the limiting factors is the time required to screen large numbers of genes. Recent advances in technology, including high-throughput methods such as microarrays, allow the screening of tens of thousands of genes (up to 30,000) in humans in a relatively short period of time.[8] To date, a limited number of published studies in schizophrenia[9–18] and in mood disorders[10, 19] have used microarrays to identify candidate genes and relevant metabolic and signaling pathways. At present, there is an early consensus of the possible role of presynaptic and myelin-related genes in the pathophysiology of schizophrenia.[15–17, 20] This review focuses on methods used in microarray technology and describes its relative strengths and weaknesses.

The central genetic dogma states that genomic DNA (Appendix 1) is first transcribed into mRNA, after which mRNA is translated into protein. Proteins are critical to a wide range of intra- and extracellular activities, including enzymatic, regulatory, and structural function. Microarrays monitor the transcriptome, the collection of mRNA in a cell. Estimates suggest that 50% of human transcriptome is expressed in the brain.[21] Changes in mRNA expression can, but not always, result in phenotypical and morphological differences. Alterations in patterns of expression of multiple genes can offer new data concerning regulatory mechanisms and biochemical pathways. Novel genes and pathways that have never been linked to the pathophysiology of psychiatric illnesses can emerge from microarray studies to provide new insight into the disease process and potential unique therapeutic drug targets.

Molecular genetic studies, in combination with the extensive new body of sequence information for the human genome, are revolutionizing the way in which cellular processes are investigated.[22] New types of experiments are possible, and discoveries are being made on an unprecedented scale. High-density DNA microarrays allow the parallel and quantitative investigation of complex mixtures of RNA and DNA (for reviews, see references 8 and 21–27).

Acquisition, Characterization, and Processing of Postmortem Brain Tissue

Table 1 summarizes the flow of the discovery process for candidate vulnerability genes with microarray technology. The first steps in the process, involving the acquisition, characterization, processing, and storage of the highest-quality brain tissue, are critical to the successful use of microarrays.[28] Major fundamental advances in psychiatry and neuroscience depend on the quality and use of brain banks. The federally funded Alzheimer's Center program has developed 29 brain banks that have been critical to its success. More than 10 brain banks focused on psychiatric disorders have been established in the United States and the United Kingdom. It is important to develop systematic standardized procedures for diagnostic reliability, clinical characterization of patients and comparison subjects, and reliable sources of tissue. Obtaining tissue, contacting next of kin for informed consent, matching patients and comparison subjects, dissecting/freezing, and processing tissue, and establishing a database, and tracking samples are important components.

Processing and Storage of Brain Tissue

Acquisition of postmortem brain tissue requires establishment of a cooperative interaction with coroner's offices, hospitals, and eye and tissue banks. Multiple daily contacts with these sources are essential to obtain postmortem material. The institutional research boards must obtain informed consent from next of kin before receiving the tissue. Once the brain tissue has been acquired, the brain can be sliced and each slice placed in a plastic envelope, photographed on each side, and flash frozen at –120°F between precooled aluminum plates. A neuropathologist should examine the tissue for abnormalities, including hemorrhage, infarcts, tumors, and plaques and tangles.

Characterization of the patients and healthy comparison subjects is particularly important and needs to include a review of the coroner's notes and psychiatric and other medical records, with all information recorded in a database. Family interviews can provide information on psychiatric symptoms, substance abuse, and family psychiatric history. Additional database information should include age, gender, postmortem interval, brain pH, manner of death, toxicology analysis, psychiat-

Table 1. Flow chart of the process for discovering candidate vulnerability genes by using microarray technology

Step	Description
1	Acquire and characterize high-quality postmortem brain tissue; match patients and comparison subjects
2	Process and store tissue
3	Dissect multiple disease-implicated brain regions
4	Extract total RNA from tissue
5	Evaluate RNA quality
6	Prepare microarrays and brain tissue samples
7	Run Affymetrix GeneChips or spotted cDNA microarrays in two independent laboratories; evaluate data and rerun samples on low-quality chips
8	Validate cellular localization of microarray results by using real-time polymerase chain reaction and in situ hybridization
9	Analyze data and statistical approaches for stringent criteria for significance of differentially expressed genes between tissue from patients and comparison subjects; compile list of candidate genes that meet criteria
10	Determine functional significance of each identified candidate gene by using web-based data review
11	Cluster genes functionally in terms of known metabolic and signaling pathways
12	Evaluate identified candidate genes in terms of their chromosomal locus and possible overlap with replicated microsatellite whole genome scan "hot spots" of mood disorder and schizophrenia patients
13	Determine overlap of the candidate gene list with genes identified in microarray studies of animals receiving psychoactive drugs
14	Redo entire experiment with new cohort of patients and matched comparison subjects

ric symptoms, substance abuse (including tobacco), age at onset of illness, and DSM-IV diagnosis. Ideally, each patient should be individually matched with important variables from healthy comparison subjects.

Regional Dissection

A great deal of information has accumulated from brain imaging (with and without pharmacological probes) and postmortem investigations to strongly implicate specific brain regions in the pathophysiology of mood disorders and schizophrenia.[29–31] For example, several articles have supported the importance of the dorsolateral prefrontal cortex in schizophrenia and the limbic system in mood disorders.[30, 32–34] A thorough literature review of these implicated regions is indicated to help determine the areas that are to be dissected from the brain. One approach is to use one side of the brain for microarray studies and the other side for parallel studies, including in situ hybridization to determine cell site specificity of the array findings. Methods have been perfected for placing frozen tissue into fixative in a manner that retains histological quality for in situ hybridization histochemistry.[35]

RNA Extraction of Total Cellular RNA From Brain Tissue and Preparation for Microarray Hybridization

Microarrays are hybridization experiments involving comparison of relative amounts of cellular mRNA from two tissue samples. The terms "hybridize" and "hybridization" mean that a single strand of DNA or RNA consisting of unpaired nucleotide bases bonds to a respective complementary nucleotide strand of DNA or RNA. Genomic DNA is usually first transcribed into mRNA in the cell nucleus and subsequently translated into proteins in the cell cytoplasm. The amount of mRNA in the cell is thought to represent the transcription of the gene. Hence, the extraction, stabilization, and purification of total RNA that includes mRNA are important factors affecting the quality of the microarray results. Total RNA is extracted from the tissue, and the quality of the total RNA is verified by electrophoresis and spectrophotometry. The mRNA is labeled and hybridized to the array for quantification. This is achieved by introducing a fluorescent marker during the preparation of mRNA that can be detected and quantified by a laser scanner.

Methods for Profiling Gene Expression

The exploitation of hybridization in microarray analyses sharply accelerated the search for defective genes. Hybridization is based on the Watson-Crick model of base pairing of nucleic acids such that adenine (A) binds to thymine (T) (or uracil [U], in the case of RNA), and cytosine (C) binds to guanine (G). Each probe on a microarray is designed to hybridize with unknown target mRNA. In this review, the term "probe" refers to known oligonucleotides (sets of short sequences of linear nucleotides) or cDNA (complementary DNA) fragments immobilized on microarray slides. (Some authors outside the oligonucleotide chip community tend to use the reverse terminology.) When samples labeled with fluorescence are applied to microarrays, hybridization or binding reactions take place between each probe and the target mRNA. Each microarray probe recognizes cDNA sequences by base pairing (hybridization). After a series of washes to eliminate unbound nucleotides and nonspecific bindings, only the target probe complexes remain bound. Intensity of the fluorescent signal for each probe reflects the abundance of the target RNA in the RNA sample.

Microarray Gene Expression Profiling

A number of functional methods for determining gene expression have been developed, including microarrays, total gene expression analysis (TOGA), massive parallel serial sequencing (MPSS), subtraction hybridization (SBF), and serial analysis of gene expression (SAGE) (SAGE is a first-pass screening method that can be used in parallel with microarrays).[36–38] This review, however, will focus on microarrays that involve synthetic oligonucleotides or complementary DNA sequences immobilized on membranes or solid surfaces.

Oligonucleotide Probe Array Method

Affymetrix GeneChip arrays (Affymetrix Inc., Santa Clara, Calif.) are high-density oligonucleotides (probes) that are synthesized on a glass slide.[22, 39] The GeneChip differs from other techniques in that the probe is generated on the slide rather than being created first and placed on the slide, as with spotted arrays. Affymetrix uses a process similar to that used in the production of solid-state semiconductors. Essentially, this method entails adding one base at a time in sequence to create the desired oligonucleotide. Synthesis involving protective chemistry and lithographic masks allows the placement of specific nucleotides in preferred locations to form multiple arrays on a single glass surface. The computer registers where each fragment or specific gene is located on the slide matrix. The known probe cDNAs that are fixed to the matrix are allowed to bind with the unknown mixture of target cDNAs. This technology allows the comparison of the expression of thousands of genes at a time between biological samples.

cDNA or Oligonucleotide Spotted Array Method

A second microarray method involves the use of robots to place or "spot" cDNA or oligonucleotides of characterized genes or ESTs (expressed sequence tags known to be expressed in the tissue but not yet characterized as genes) nucleotide sequences to a slide or membrane. The genetic material to be identified (cDNA or oligonucleotides) is washed over and allowed to hybridize to the spotted arrays, after which it is excited with lasers to activate a fluorescent signal. Scanning confocal microscopes measure the signal intensities of the hybridization. The measurements are then translated into ratios to provide relative comparisons of mRNA from different samples. The strength of the spotted arrays is that they can be customized to measure different mRNA variants.

Robots are used to control the position and spotting of the cDNA or oligonucleotides. This produces accurate high-density arrays. With this method, experimental and reference samples are typically labeled with red or green fluorochrome. Both are hybridized on the same microarray, and a measurement is obtained from each DNA site on the array. The intensity differences of the two fluorescent images are read out as differences in gene transcript abundance between the experimental and reference tissue (patient brain tissue and healthy comparison tissue). Radioactively labeled targets may also be used.[40] Several companies such as CodeLink[41] have developed spotted oligonucleotide microarrays consisting of nucleotide (50–80-nucleotide) probes.

Strengths of Microarrays

The strength of microarrays is that they provide the means to repeatedly measure the expression levels of a large number of genes at a time. Relatively small amounts of total RNA can be analyzed.

Limitations of Microarrays

Microarrays are primarily a screening tool. Although traditional methods that measure gene expression (e.g., Northern blotting, RNase protection assays) are relatively labor intensive, they provide high resolution and can be used to validate or extend microarray data. Several limitations to microarrays are noted. A major limitation is a decreased sensitivity of the arrays to the detection of genes with low expression levels (low-abundance genes). Another disadvantage is that microarrays do not measure posttranslational modifications (e.g., phosphorylation).[21] Still another drawback is that it is possible to confound microarray results through a process of cross-hybridization in which specific components of the arrays will cross-hybridize because of sequence similarity of the probes as defined by Affymetrix. This is actually more of a problem with spotted DNA arrays since there is no attempt to spot onto the arrays only the portions of genes that are different from their family members. Affymetrix can, in principle, avoid this problem by using oligos corresponding to only the regions that differ in sequence between closely related genes. Finally, tissue heterogeneity remains a persistent challenge for microarray studies, particularly in brains in which there are multiple densely packed cell types. This is also true for Northern blots, SAGE, and any other non-in-situ method. Microarray measures of heterogeneous cell expression may decrease the sensitivity of microarrays by masking changes in gene expression.[42] To overcome this problem, laser-capture microdissection techniques are used that can measure the expression of single cells, providing the capability of isolating homogenous samples from heterogeneous blocks of tissue.[42] Microarrays and laser-capture microdissection, used in parallel, provide complementary information concerning cell-specific gene expression changes representative of larger blocks of tissue.

Verification of Quality of mRNA

It is necessary to optimize the integrity of RNA, especially in studies of the postmortem brain. In this regard, pre- and postagonal status should be recorded. It has been generally agreed that the preservation of mRNA is affected by its preagonal state. Coma, pyrexia, and hypoxia are considered to affect specific mRNA. mRNA is preserved for long periods in postmortem tissue, and the postmortem interval (time from death until freezing of the tissue) has little effect on the stability of RNA for at least 48 hours. Since the preservation of mRNA correlates with brain pH, measurement of brain tissue pH is considered to be a useful initial screening procedure in the assessment of samples.[43, 44] Longer postmortem intervals do not appear to affect brain pH (data in preparation).

The evaluation of RNA sample quality is essential for interpreting microarray results. In experiments using Affymetrix GeneChips, 3':5' ratios (ratios of signal intensities of probes designed specifically for each end region of a gene) of housekeeping genes (genes whose expression is essential for cell function) are useful as indicators of mRNA integrity in the genes. The percentage of present call (percentage of genes detected as present in samples of total genes on the microarray) can also be used in evaluating RNA integrity in microarray experiments. When there is a problem in either RNA integrity or in another part of the microarray experiment, the percent of present call is detected as low. Correlation between arrays can be a particularly sensitive indicator for

RNA integrity (data in preparation). On the basis of our analyses, arrays from samples with better RNA integrity correlate better with each other.

Additional variables need to be considered in microarray methods. Repeated freezing and thawing of RNA samples leads to degradation of the sample. Storage of RNA samples at below –70°C is essential. Conversion of samples to cDNA, rather than maintaining samples as RNA for a long time, will aid in the preservation of samples rather than maintaining samples as RNA for a long time.

Other microarray quality-control parameters include the use of multiple array experiments to eliminate noise in the data (e.g., technical duplicates in which the sample is relabeled and hybridized to a new chip) or biological replicates. Similarity of expression profiles of replicate experiments helps to validate the quality of the study. All samples not meeting rigorous standards for high-quality data should be rerun.

Validation and Localization

Microarray methods are essentially for screening, and results obtained from them need to be validated. In situ hybridization (ISH) histochemistry provides one of the important confirmations of the expression of genes in the brain and can be used at multiple levels of resolution to confirm the presence of relevant mRNA in a region of the CNS, its localization to subnuclei or layers, and the classes of cells in which it is expressed. In determining cell class, it is important to have tissue in a sufficiently well-preserved state to permit immunocytochemistry. Radioactive in situ hybridization histochemistry can be applied in a quantitative manner to confirm expression levels demonstrated by array studies and can be used to quantify numbers of neurons in cases in which the concentration of signal over cell somata is sufficiently dense and well localized (see examples of both in references 45 and 46). The limiting factor for in situ hybridization studies is the time taken to prepare oligonucleotide or complementary RNA probes for novel mRNA and the concentrated effort required to do in situ runs on multiple candidates.

Real-Time Polymerase Chain Reaction

Real-time polymerase chain reaction (RT-PCR) is another relatively high-throughput technique used for the quantification of steady-state mRNA levels. It provides high sensitivity so that rare sequences can be detected. It may also be used to detect messages from small sections of tissue so that subsections of the brain can be examined independently. Real-time polymerase chain reaction involves polymerase chain reaction amplification of a segment of the gene from mRNA that has been turned into cDNA and measurement by fluorescence of the polymerase chain reaction product formed by interactions of a green dye with the double-stranded DNA product. This method is sensitive and inexpensive.

Other real-time polymerase chain reaction methods, such as the Taq-Man probe assay (Applied Biosystems, Foster City, Calif.) with fluorescent-labeled probes, have been developed. These technologies increase specificity of real-time polymerase chain reaction detections by way of mechanisms that activate the fluorescent signal only when the fluorescent-labeled probe is specifically bound to a target sequence.

SAGE: An Alternative to Microarray Methods

In psychiatry, there is a strong incentive to use SAGE to complement microarrays, both in terms of dealing with the sensitivity limitations of microarrays and the need to identify novel transcripts. The SAGE method is designed to produce estimates of the relative concentration of the mRNA pool in a tissue. This high-throughput strategy uses sequencing of short fragments of mRNA on a large scale (many tens of thousands to hundreds of thousands of such RNA pieces are thereby uniquely identified). It is largely seen as a means of gene expression profiling for a tissue both to determine if a tissue makes an mRNA and in the quantification of each RNA.[36, 47] The SAGE method can be used to quantify various mRNAs in a tissue; however, it can require pooling tissue blocks across individuals (in order to be able to build a library large enough to detect rare mRNAs). SAGE is also very expensive. Advantages include that it does not require knowing all the transcripts beforehand, as in the case of microarrays. In one recent study, SAGE was used to evaluate the sensitivity of Affymetrix U95a human chips. It is estimated that GeneChips reliably detect 30% of hippocampal transcriptome when a gross hippocampal dissection is used as the source tissue.[47]

Bioinformatics

Defining Criteria for Significance of Identified Genes

New methods of data analysis are being developed to efficiently process the massive amount of data produced by microarray studies. Systematic mathematical strategies that can be applied to large numbers of research designs become critical to correctly handle the extraordinarily large data sets. There are three algorithms in current use for oligonucleotide microarray expression analysis: MAS5 (Microarray Suite version 5, Affymetrix), dCHIP,[48] and RMA (Robust Microarray Analysis).[49] These software packages condense the 20 Affymetrix probe pairs of a set, corresponding to each gene, into one value. Whatever package is used, the resulting condensed value can then be used for later statistical analyses.

With a simple two-group comparison, a t test or a Wilcoxon test is commonly used as a statistical indicator of the effect size. However, both tests have limitations in that multiple tests (thousands of observed genes) are usually performed for each sample, thus raising the possibility of false discovery, and the t test must be repeated for multiple group comparisons, increasing the number of statistical tests performed. To minimize the false positive and false negative discovery of candidate genes in a microarray, other selection criteria can be implemented, such as coupling a fold change (ratio of experimental gene expression divided by comparison gene expression) and statistical requirement together. Often investigators use signal intensity, assuming some proportionality to gene abundance, as another criterion for selection of genes to follow up for validation, functional, or structural studies.

A regression approach can be useful when evaluating differences between group means for gene expression (especially when more than two groups are being compared) and when there is consideration of variables such as diagnosis, gender, and brain region. Covariates can be built into regression analyses by using age, family history, agonal factors, and tissue factors such as pH, postmortem interval, and time to cooling of the tissue. During evaluation of more than two groups, a simple regression approach through an analysis of variance procedure is useful for incorporating repeated measurements obtained from the same sample (technical duplicate) and from different brain regions of the same patient. Currently, microarray statistical analysis software is freely available through academic ventures such as BioConductor (http://www. bioconductor.org).

Interpretation of Changes in Gene Expression

Microarrays have traditionally used fold change (the ratio of experimental gene expression divided by comparison gene expression) as an index of the magnitude of differences in gene expression between samples.[50] Many factors, including data standardization and the abundance of genes, may confound fold change; therefore, other rigorous statistical approaches (see Bioinformatics) are necessary in addition to fold-change measurements.[48, 50, 51] When a set of genes is identified by microarray experiments (i.e., stringently and significantly differentiated from matched comparison subjects), it is useful to describe each gene in terms of its chromosomal locus, functions, effects of psychoactive drugs, and significance in psychiatric disorders. Also needed is information about the similarity of gene sequences between human and animal genomes. Perhaps most important is the issue of whether the gene is involved in specific known metabolic or signaling pathways. What other genes are interacting with the gene of interest? Are other genes in the pathway also differentially expressed? Most microarrays contain a specific number of genes that can be categorized in 40 or more defined metabolic or signaling pathways.

Additional information is gained from microarray analysis of multiple brain regions, including data concerning whether classes of genes are globally dysregulated in many areas or only in a particular region. Analyzing multiple brain regions in two independent laboratories can serve to reduce false experiment-wide error rates, since the entire experiment is essentially replicated with multiple biological samples.

Functional Significance of Genes in Terms of Metabolic and Signaling Pathways

Once the task of identifying candidate genes is completed, the process of delineating the biological significance of the observed differential gene expression patterns begins. It involves identifying the function of individual genes or their products, clustering them to reveal their relation to each other and predicting functions of gene clusters with previously unknown functions, deducing their causal relationship to the disease under study, and defining the biochemical mechanism/pathway they could likely disrupt or through which they exert their influence and/or participate in the disease process (GO project [http://www.geneontology.org]). The functional attributes of each known gene or gene product (protein) fall into three basic categories: 1) molecular function (e.g., growth factor), 2) cellular components (cellular location) (e.g., cytoskeleton), and 3) biological process (physiological pathway) (e.g., energy metabolism) (Gene Ontology Consortium 2000). Many additional sources of relevant information are available, including the National Center for Biotechnology Information (NCBI) (http://www.ncbi.nlm.nih.gov), the NINDS/NIMH Microarray Consortium (http://arrayconsortium.cnmcresearch.org), and the German Genome Resource Center (http://www.rzpd.de).

Changes in Gene Expression Due to Medication and Epigenetic Factors

Psychoactive medication can have a significant influence on genes associated with signaling and metabolic pathways. It is important to determine which medications patients have received, their dose, lifetime exposure, and the medications taken at the time of death. The potential alterations in gene expression in postmortem brain tissue due to psychoactive drugs can be evaluated with microarray studies in rodents and nonhuman primates receiving long-term doses of medications. Epigenetic processes can be also evaluated in terms of their impact on expression changes for a given gene.

Identifying Candidate Vulnerability Genes

The top section of Figure 1 summarizes a strategy for discovering candidate vulnerability genes. Microarrays provide a unique high-throughput methodology for identifying a set of significant genes that are differentially expressed in psychiatric subjects in relation to matched comparison subjects. These genes can be validated with real-time polymerase chain reactions and their cellular location identified by in situ hybridization studies. One can then review replicated genome-wide survey-identified "hot spots" and genes located in these regions of interest. Although a number of genes occur at these hot-spot loci, the microarray-identified genes that are found at these loci may be of particular interest. A third source of candidate genes comes from the use of microarrays in animal models of psychiatric disease. For example, behavioral paradigms such as learned helplessness and the forced swim test[52] and drug treatment models in which animals are administered phencyclidine,[53] amphetamine,[40, 54, 55] or long-term treatment with antidepressants, mood stabilizers,[56–58] or typical or atypical neuroleptics[20] provide important resources for microarray studies in psychiatric illness. It is possible to develop Venn diagrams to define genes that are similarly differentially expressed, for example, in all three classes of mood stabilizers (e.g., lithium, valproate, or carbamazepine). Finally, candidate vulnerability genes can be derived from our knowledge of the pathophysiology of circuits, neurotransmitter systems, and the pharmacology of the disease. Genes become candidates of major interest when they are 1) identified by microarray screens in patient postmortem brain tissue, 2) occur on replicated whole genome-wide hot spots, 3) are implicated in diseased rodent or nonhuman primate models, and 4) relate to metabolic or signaling pathways known to be involved in the disease.

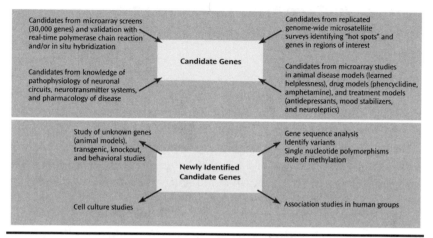

Figure 1. Process for discovery of candidate vulnerability genes and their biological investigation

The top section of Figure 1 summarizes a strategy for discovering candidate vulnerability genes. When a gene is identified as a potential candidate, studies move to the next stage of biological validation (bottom section).

Investigative Analyses of Candidate Vulnerability Genes

When a gene is identified as a potential candidate, studies move to the next stage of biological validation (Figure 1, bottom section). Further efforts in the investigation involve multiple strategies for studying structure and gene function. In some cases, the gene in question is a well-known one, and the fundamental question is whether it is contributing to the disease process because of alterations of its structure or in its level of expression. In other cases, the gene is either totally unknown or can be assigned to a general class of gene families but without direct evidence of its biological role. In such cases, beyond addressing the potential structural questions, one needs to begin to address its function. One approach involves tissue culture strategies. Ascertaining the functional role of a given gene by using transgenic or knockout animal models represents an ultimate test of its hypothesized role.

Gene-sequence analysis can be conducted in an attempt to identify single nucleotide polymorphisms (SNPs), variations that occur in human DNA, in the coding or in the promoter domain of the gene, splice variations, or actual mutations. By using BLAST (Basic Local Alignment Search Tool, National Center for Biotechnology Information, Bethesda, Md.), one can search the existing databases for genes with sequence similarity in human and other published animal genomes. This information may greatly help identify important functions of the gene.[59]

Tissue Culture Strategies

Cell culture studies have been heavily used to evaluate the function of mRNA that is seen as interesting in microarray studies. This approach to understanding the biology of mRNA has considerable value, yet can be expensive, limited to certain cell types, and may reveal only a fraction of that mRNA's function across cells or in an organ. However, a careful analysis may open many doors to a functional view of the effects of activation or inhibition of a gene, its mRNA, and the protein derived from it. This is especially true if the functions of the gene and its products are not known except for their sequences. The tissue culture expression of an mRNA and its derived protein is a good step into biology and may then lead to other studies, such as transgenic animals, knock-ins, and knockouts of this mRNA's gene.

Animal Models

Using microarrays to learn the pattern of gene expression in the brain (and other tissues) is a first and critical step. Substantially different hypotheses can then evolve from in situ hybridization studies, revealing a pattern that demonstrates expression in every cell versus a subset of cells. For example, a gene that is neuronal and is primarily expressed in the extended amygdala may lead us to hypotheses about a role in emotional reactivity, whereas a gene that is present at all synapses may lead to hypotheses relating to signaling or synaptic plasticity. The neuronal site expression pattern will then guide the choice of animal models to be pursued. For example, a gene highly expressed in emotional circuits will call for studies using models of anxiety-like behaviors (the elevated-plus maze, light-dark box, fear conditioning). By contrast, a gene highly expressed in the hippocampus might suggest a possible role in learning and memory (e.g., the radial-arm maze or Morris water maze).

A powerful strategy for investigating the function of a given gene is the use of transgenic and knockout mice. These approaches involve artificial interference with the level of expression of a gene in an organism, ranging from completely eliminating expression (knockout) to significant overexpression by using a transgenic approach. These tools are intrinsically very demanding in that they require the production, char-

Table 2.   Investigations of the function and structure of candidate genes following identification by microarray technology

Step	Description
1	Review web-based data sequence for similarity of candidate genes to the human genome and other completed animal genomes for clues concerning functional and metabolic and signaling pathways
2	Examine effects of known and unknown identified genes in transgenic and knockout animal studies
3	Examine cell culture studies for candidate gene function
4	Analyze structure of candidate genes and identify sequence variants, including single nucleotide polymorphisms (SNPs) in promoter and exon regions
5	Consider microarray studies of single cells in selected brain regions using laser capture microdissection to increase homogeneity of the RNA sample source
6	Consider association studies in human groups
7	Use these newly identified genes as unique targets for therapeutic drug development for schizophrenia and mood disorders

acterization, and maintenance of novel lines of mice. However, these approaches, if properly used, can reveal gene functions that cannot be elucidated by means of any of the nongenetic approaches. There have been significant improvements of these techniques that have resulted in enhanced control over the regional specificity of the gene expression as well as the timing of the altered expression.[60–62] Control over timing and spatial expression substantially increases the ability to deduce the functions of the candidate gene. Together, this combination of tools allows a group of investigators to move a particular gene from a candidate with altered expression associated with an illness to a specific target with much better characterization of patterns of neural expression, regulation, and function. Table 2 summarizes postarray investigations, including the function and structure of identified candidate genes.

Future Developments

1. In the near future, DNA microarrays will provide a method for simultaneously monitoring levels of nearly every gene transcript in the human genome. This is particularly useful in the mammalian brain, which is divided into many anatomically distinct regions. Affymetrix has used information from the draft of the human genome to design arrays (U133) that contain 39,000 gene transcripts.

2. Advances in spotted DNA arrays include the greater availability and quality of full-length cDNA clones for spotting on chips. Longer oligonucleotides are also starting to be used with standard spotting technology.
3. Other new applications of microarrays involve the study of binding sites for transcription factors on a genome-wide level.[8]
4. New discoveries in combinatorial chemical processing promise to advance microarray technology. These include new digital light processors and simplified synthesis of nucleic acids.[25]

In summary, data from microarray experiments can provide powerful information to help determine the causes of psychiatric illness, the mechanisms by which psychoactive drugs work, and what gene products may be unique targets for therapy in these disorders.

Appendix 1.   Glossary of selected genetic terms

DNA   (deoxyribonucleic acid) carrier of inherited information; DNA makes RNA, and RNA makes protein

cDNA   (complementary DNA) a copy of DNA

hybridize   to bind complementary base pairs of DNA molecules

in situ hybridization   a hybridization procedure to confirm the presence of relevant mRNAs and define the localization and cell class

knockout   eliminating expression of a gene, usually in a mouse

mRNA   (messenger RNA) translated into protein

nucleotides   basic subunits of DNA

oligonucleotides   short linear stretches of nucleotides

probe   in this review, probe refers to the known cDNA or oligonucleotides affixed to the array surface

real-time polymerase chain reaction   a high-throughput method to quantify mRNA levels

RNA   (ribonucleic acid) a molecule that is formed as an intermediate between DNA and protein in the process of gene expression

SNPs   (single nucleotide polymorphisms) variations that occur in human DNA

target   in this review, target refers to the labeled unknown material that is bound to the cDNA or oligonucleotide on the array

transcript   mRNA that encodes a protein

transcription   the process of copying DNA into RNA

transcriptome   all expressed mRNA in a cell

transgenic   producing overexpression of a gene, usually in a mouse

translation   synthesis of protein from RNA

References

1. Sawa A, Snyder SH: Schizophrenia: diverse approaches to a complex disease. Science 2002; 296:692–695
2. Mowry BJ, Nancarrow DJ: Molecular genetics of schizophrenia. Clin Exp Pharmacol Physiol 2001; 28:66–69
3. Nemeroff CB, Owens MJ: Treatment of mood disorders. Nat Neurosci 2002; 5(Nov suppl):1068–1070
4. Tandon R, Jibson MD: Efficacy of newer generation antipsychotics in the treatment of schizophrenia. Psychoneuroendocrinology 2003; 28(suppl 1):9–26
5. Kato C, Petronis A, Okazaki Y, Tochigi M, Umekage T, Sasaki T: Molecular genetic studies of schizophrenia: challenges and insights. Neurosci Res 2002; 43:295–304
6. Avissar S, Schreiber G: Toward molecular diagnostics of mood disorders in psychiatry. Trends Mol Med 2002; 8:294–300
7. Johnston-Wilson NL, Bouton CM, Pevsner J, Breen JJ, Torrey EF, Yolken RH: Emerging technologies for large-scale screening of human tissues and fluids in the study of severe psychiatric disease. Int J Neuropsychopharmacol 2001; 4:83–92
8. Shoemaker DD, Linsley PS: Recent developments in DNA microarrays. Curr Opin Microbiol 2002; 5:334–337
9. Novak G, Kim D, Seeman P, Tallerico T: Schizophrenia and Nogo: elevated mRNA in cortex, and high prevalence of a homozygous CAA insert. Brain Res Mol Brain Res 2002; 107:183–189
10. Mimmack ML, Ryan M, Baba H, Navarro-Ruiz J, Iritani S, Faull RL, McKenna PJ, Jones PB, Arai H, Starkey M, Emson PC, Bahn S: Gene expression analysis in schizophrenia: reproducible up-regulation of several members of the apolipoprotein L family located in a high-susceptibility locus for schizophrenia on chromosome 22. Proc Natl Acad Sci USA 2002; 99:4680–4685
11. Middleton FA, Mirnics K, Pierri JN, Lewis DA, Levitt P: Gene expression profiling reveals alterations of specific metabolic pathways in schizophrenia. J Neurosci 2002; 22:2718–2729
12. Vawter MP, Barrett T, Cheadle C, Sokolov BP, Wood WH III, Donovan DM, Webster M, Freed WJ, Becker KG: Application of cDNA microarrays to examine gene expression differences in schizophrenia. Brain Res Bull 2001; 55:641–650
13. Mirnics K, Middleton FA, Lewis DA, Levitt P: Analysis of complex brain disorders with gene expression microarrays: schizophrenia as a disease of the synapse. Trends Neurosci 2001; 24:479–486
14. Mirnics K, Middleton FA, Stanwood GD, Lewis DA, Levitt P: Disease-specific changes in regulator of G-protein signaling 4 (RGS4) expression in schizophrenia. Mol Psychiatry 2001; 6:293–301

15. Vawter MP, Crook JM, Hyde TM, Kleinman JE, Weinberger DR, Becker KG, Freed WJ: Microarray analysis of gene expression in the prefrontal cortex in schizophrenia: a preliminary study. Schizophr Res 2002; 58:11–20

16. Hakak Y, Walker JR, Li C, Wong WH, Davis KL, Buxbaum JD, Haroutunian V, Fienberg AA: Genome-wide expression analysis reveals dysregulation of myelination-related genes in chronic schizophrenia. Proc Natl Acad Sci USA 2001; 98:4746–4751

17. Hof PR, Haroutunian V, Copland C, Davis KL, Buxbaum JD: Molecular and cellular evidence for an oligodendrocyte abnormality in schizophrenia. Neurochem Res 2002; 27:1193–1200

18. Wurmbach E, Gonzalez-Maeso J, Yuen T, Ebersole BJ, Mastaitis JW, Mobbs CV, Sealfon SC: Validated genomic approach to study differentially expressed genes in complex tissues. Neurochem Res 2002; 27:1027–1033

19. Bezchlibnyk YB, Wang JF, McQueen GM, Young LT: Gene expression differences in bipolar disorder revealed by cDNA array analysis of postmortem frontal cortex. J Neurochem 2001; 79:826–834

20. Mirnics K, Middleton FA, Marquez A, Lewis DA, Levitt P: Molecular characterization of schizophrenia viewed by microarray analysis of gene expression in prefrontal cortex. Neuron 2000; 28:53–67

21. Luo Z, Geschwind DH: Microarray applications in neuroscience. Neurobiol Dis 2001; 8:183–193

22. Lockhart DJ, Winzeler EA: Genomics, gene expression and DNA arrays. Nature 2000; 405:827–836

23. Watson SJ, Meng F, Thompson RC, Akil H: The "chip" as a specific genetic tool. Biol Psychiatry 2000; 48:1147–1156

24. Watson SJ, Akil H: Gene chips and arrays revealed: a primer on their power and their uses. Biol Psychiatry 1999; 45:533–543

25. Pongrac J, Middleton FA, Lewis DA, Levitt P, Mirnics K: Gene expression profiling with DNA microarrays: advancing our understanding of psychiatric disorders. Neurochem Res 2002; 27:1049–1063

26. Cowan WM, Kopnisky KL, Hyman SE: The human genome project and its impact on psychiatry. Annu Rev Neurosci 2002; 25:1–50

27. Shilling PD, Kelsoe JR: Functional genomics approaches to understanding brain disorders. Pharmacogenomics 2002; 3:31–45

28. Akbarian S, Kim JJ, Potkin SG, Hetrick WP, Bunney WE Jr, Jones EG: Maldistribution of interstitial neurons in prefrontal white matter of the brains of schizophrenic patients. Arch Gen Psychiatry 1996; 53:425–436

29. Dunn RT, Kimbrell TA, Ketter TA, Frye MA, Willis MW, Luckenbaugh DA, Post RM: Principal components of the Beck Depression Inventory and regional cerebral metabolism in unipolar and bipolar depression. Biol Psychiatry 2002; 51:387–399

30. Bunney WE, Bunney BG: Evidence for a compromised dorsolateral prefrontal cortical parallel circuit in schizophrenia. Brain Res Brain Res Rev 2000; 31:138–146

31. Ketter TA, George MS, Kimbress TA, Willis MW, Benson BE, Post RM: Neuroanatomical models and brain imaging studies, in Bipolar Disorder: Biological Models and Their Clinical Applications. Edited by Young LT, Joffe RT. New York, Marcel Dekker, 1997, pp 179–217

32. Wu J, Buchsbaum MS, Gillin JC, Tang C, Cadwell S, Keator D, Fallon JH, Wiegand M, Najafi A, Klein E, Hazen K, Bunney WE Jr: Prediction of antidepressant effects of sleep deprivation by metabolic rates in the ventral anterior cingulate and medial prefrontal cortex. Am J Psychiatry 1999; 156:1149–1158; correction, 156:1666

33. Mayberg HS: Limbic-cortical dysregulation: a proposed model of depression. J Neuropsychiatry Clin Neurosci 1997; 9:471–481

34. Tamminga CA, Vogel M, Gao X, Lahti AC, Holcomb HH: The limbic cortex in schizophrenia: focus on the anterior cingulate. Brain Res Brain Res Rev 2000; 31:364–370

35. Jones EG, Hendry SH, Liu XB, Hodgins S, Potkin SG, Tourtellotte WW: A method for fixation of previously fresh-frozen human adult and fetal brains that preserves histological quality and immunoreactivity. J Neurosci Methods 1992; 44:133–144

36. Velculescu VE: Essay: Amersham Pharmacia Biotech and Science Prize: tantalizing transcriptomes—SAGE and its use in global gene expression analysis. Science 1999; 286:1491–1492

37. Sutcliffe JG, Foye PE, Erlander MG, Hilbush BS, Bodzin LJ, Durham JT, Hasel KW: TOGA: an automated parsing technology for analyzing expression of nearly all genes. Proc Natl Acad Sci USA 2000; 97:1976–1981

38. Brenner S, Johnson M, Bridgham J, Golda G, Lloyd DH, Johnson D, Luo S, McCurdy S, Foy M, Ewan M, Roth R, George D, Eletr S, Albrecht G, Vermaas E, Williams SR, Moon K, Burcham T, Pallas M, DuBridge RB, Kirchner J, Fearon K, Mao J, Corcoran K: Gene expression analysis by massively parallel signature sequencing (MPSS) on microbead arrays. Nat Biotechnol 2000; 18:630–634

39. Lipshutz RJ, Fodor SP, Gingeras TR, Lockhart DJ: High-density synthetic oligonucleotide arrays. Nat Genet 1999; 21(1 suppl):20–24

40. Barrett T, Xie T, Piao Y, Dillon-Carter O, Kargul GJ, Lim MK, Chrest FJ, Wersto R, Rowley DL, Juhaszova M, Zhou L, Vawter MP, Becker KG, Cheadle C, Wood WH III, McCann UD, Freed WJ, Ko MS, Ricaurte GA, Donovan DM: A murine dopamine neuron-specific cDNA library and microarray: increased COX1 expression during methamphetamine neurotoxicity. Neurobiol Dis 2001; 8:822–833

41. Ramakrishnan R, Dorris D, Lublinsky A, Nguyen A, Domanus M, Prokhorova A, Gieser L, Touma E, Lockner R, Tata M, Zhu X, Patterson M, Shippy R, Sendera TJ, Mazumder A: An assessment of Motorola CodeLink

microarray performance for gene expression profiling applications. Nucleic Acids Res 2002; 30(7):e30

42. Torres-Munoz J, Stockton P, Tacoronte N, Roberts B, Maronpot RR, Petito CK: Detection of HIV-1 gene sequences in hippocampal neurons isolated from postmortem AIDS brains by laser capture microdissection. J Neuropathol Exp Neurol 2001; 60:885–892

43. Kingsbury AE, Foster OJ, Nisbet AP, Cairns N, Bray L, Eve DJ, Lees AJ, Marsden CD: Tissue pH as an indicator of mRNA preservation in human post-mortem brain. Brain Res Mol Brain Res 1995; 28:311–318

44. Barton AJ, Pearson RC, Najlerahim A, Harrison PJ: Pre- and postmortem influences on brain RNA. J Neurochem 1993; 61:1–11

45. Akbarian S, Kim JJ, Potkin SG, Hagman JO, Tafazzoli A, Bunney WE Jr, Jones EG: Gene expression for glutamic acid decarboxylase is reduced without loss of neurons in prefrontal cortex of schizophrenics. Arch Gen Psychiatry 1995; 52:258–266

46. Akbarian S, Sucher NJ, Bradley D, Tafazzoli A, Trinh D, Hetrick WP, Potkin SG, Sandman CA, Bunney WE Jr, Jones EG: Selective alterations in gene expression for NMDA receptor subunits in prefrontal cortex of schizophrenics. J Neurosci 1996; 16:19–30

47. Evans SJ, Datson NA, Kabbaj M, Thompson RC, Vreugdenhil E, De Kloet ER, Watson SJ, Akil H: Evaluation of Affymetrix Gene Chip sensitivity in rat hippocampal tissue using SAGE (serial analysis of gene expression) analysis. Eur J Neurosci 2002; 16:409–413

48. Li C, Hung Wong W: Model-based analysis of oligonucleotide arrays: model validation, design issues and standard error application. Genome Biol 2001; 2(8):RESEARCH0032

49. Irizarry RA, Hobbs B, Collins F, Beazer-Barclay YD, Antonellis KJ, Scherf U, Speed TP: Exploration, normalization, and summaries of high-density oligonucleotide array probe level data. http://biosun01.biostat.jhsph.edu/~ririzarr/papers/affy1.pdf

50. Draghici S: Statistical intelligence: effective analysis of high-density microarray data. Drug Discov Today 2002; 7:S55–S63

51. Yang YH, Speed T: Design issues for cDNA microarray experiments. Nat Rev Genet 2002; 3:579–588

52. Nestler EJ, Gould E, Manji H, Buncan M, Duman RS, Greshenfeld HK, Hen R, Koester S, Lederhendler I, Meaney M, Robbins T, Winsky L, Zalcman S: Preclinical models: status of basic research in depression. Biol Psychiatry 2002; 52:503–528

53. Joo A, Shibata H, Ninomiya H, Kawasaki H, Tashiro N, Fukumaki Y: Structure and polymorphisms of the human metabotropic glutamate receptor type 2 gene (GRM2): analysis of association with schizophrenia. Mol Psychiatry 2001; 6:186–192

54. Niculescu AB III, Segal DS, Kuczenski R, Barrett T, Hauger RL, Kelsoe JR: Identifying a series of candidate genes for mania and psychosis: a convergent functional genomics approach. Physiol Genomics 2000; 4:83–91

55. Niculescu AB III, Kelsoe JR: The human genome: genetic testing and animal models (image, neuro). Am J Psychiatry 2001; 158:1587

56. Bosetti F, Seemann R, Bell JM, Zahorchak R, Friedman E, Rapoport SI, Manickam P: Analysis of gene expression with cDNA microarrays in rat brain after 7 and 42 days of oral lithium administration. Brain Res Bull 2002; 57:205–209

57. Yamada M, Yamazaki S, Takahashi K, Nara K, Ozawa H, Yamada S, Kiuchi Y, Oguchi K, Kamijima K, Higuchi T, Momose K: Induction of cysteine string protein after chronic antidepressant treatment in rat frontal cortex. Neurosci Lett 2001; 301:183–186

58. Manji HK, Chen G: PKC, MAP kinases and the bcl-2 family of proteins as long-term targets for mood stabilizers. Mol Psychiatry 2002; 7(suppl 1):S46–S56

59. Pennacchio LA, Olivier M, Hubacek JA, Cohen JC, Cox DR, Fruchart JC, Krauss RM, Rubin EM: An apolipoprotein influencing triglycerides in humans and mice revealed by comparative sequencing. Science 2001; 294:169–173

60. Tsien JZ, Chen DF, Gerber D, Tom C, Mercer EH, Anderson DJ, Mayford M, Kandel ER, Tonegawa S: Subregion- and cell type-restricted gene knockout in mouse brain. Cell 1996; 87:1317–1326

61. Mayford M, Bach ME, Huang YY, Wang L, Hawkins RD, Kandel ER: Control of memory formation through regulated expression of a CaMKII transgene. Science 1996; 274:1678–1683

62. DePrato Primeaux S, Holmes PV, Martin RJ, Dean RG, Edwards GL: Experimentally induced attenuation of neuropeptide-Y gene expression in transgenic mice increases mortality rate following seizures. Neurosci Lett 2000; 287:61–64

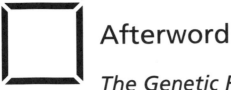

Afterword

The Genetic Revolution: The Importance of Flies and Worms

It seems remarkable that within 50 years of the discovery of the double helical structure of DNA, the genetic code was deciphered, recombinant DNA technology was devised, and the nucleotide sequences of the entire genomes of man, mouse, the fruit fly (*Drosophila*), the nematode (*Caenorhabditis elegans*), yeast, and many other organisms were determined. The discovery of thousands of genes represents one of the great achievements of science, yet the functions of most genes remain unknown. Eventually, it will surely be found that some of these genes are involved in psychiatric or neurological diseases. A tremendous opportunity exists to explore the functions of these genes by various means, including mutation or RNA interference. The latter method depends on the use of double-stranded RNA, or oligoribonucleotides, to temporarily destroy the corresponding species of mRNA, thereby resulting in a temporary mutant phenotype.

Comparative genomics has shown that *Drosophila* and *C. elegans* have many genes for proteins involved in neural information processing that are similar to genes found in humans. Thirty-eight genes that bear some similarity to genes thought to be involved in human neurological diseases have been found in *Drosophila*, including parkin, β-amyloid precursor–like protein, presenilin, tau (involved in frontotemporal dementia with parkinsonism), and neuroserpin (involved in familial encephalopathy);[1]some genes have also been found in *C. elegans*. There are many advantages to studying such genes in *Drosophila* or *C. elegans*, since many genetic techniques are available that can be

---

[1]Rubin GM, et al: Comparative genomics of the eukaryotes. Science 2000; 287:2204–2215

used to investigate the functions of proteins, whereas similar studies in the mouse would be too time consuming or expensive to be feasible. For example, to find compounds that enhance memory in humans, hundreds of thousands of compounds are being screened currently in *Drosophila* by Timothy Tully of Cold Spring Harbor Laboratory.

Thus, the revolution in molecular genetics has created tremendous opportunities to do research that surely will lead to fundamental advances in knowledge of normal and pathological processes in psychiatry and neurobiology. But only in the human can one explore the psychological and social factors that influence behavior.

Marshall Nirenberg, Ph.D.

Index

Page numbers printed in **boldface** type refer to tables or figures.